# Italian Cooking

## 130 Authentic Homemade Italian Recipes That Are Quick & Easy to Cook (And That the Whole Family Will LOVE)!

by Olivia Rogers

Copyright © 2017 By Olivia Rogers
All rights reserved. No part of this book may be reproduced in any form without permission in writing from the author. No part of this publication may be reproduced or transmitted in any form or by any means, mechanic, electronic, photocopying, recording, by any storage or retrieval system, or transmitted by email without the permission in writing from the author and publisher.
For information regarding permissions write to author at
Olivia@TheMenuAtHome.com
Reviewers may quote brief passages in review.

Please note that credit for the images used in this book go to the respective owners.
You can view this at: TheMenuAtHome.com/image-list

Olivia Rogers
TheMenuAtHome.com

## Table of Contents

*Introduction* _____ 9
*1. Pizza Margherita* _____ 9
*2. Spicy Sausage & Mushroom Pizza* _____ 11
*3. Bacon, Tomato & Arugula Pizza* _____ 12
*4. Chicken & Herb White Pizza* _____ 13
*5. Four-Cheese Pizza* _____ 15
*6. Garlicky Clam Grilled Pizza* _____ 18
*7. Smoked Salmon Thin-Crust Pizza* _____ 19
*8. Pepperoni Deep-Dish Pizza* _____ 21
*9. Veggie Grilled Pizza* _____ 22
*10. Quick Pizza Margherita* _____ 24
*11. Greek Lamb Pizza* _____ 25
*12. Arugula Pizza with Poached Eggs* _____ 25
*13. Peach & Gorgonzola Chicken Pizza* _____ 27
*14. Roasted Vegetable & Ricotta Pizza* _____ 28
*15. Artichoke & Arugula Pizza with Prosciutto* _____ 29
*16. Supreme Pizza* _____ 30
*17. Apricot & Prosciutto Thin-Crust Pizza* _____ 31
*18. Rustic Pasta Toss* _____ 33
*19. Italian Tilapia Parmesan with Pasta* _____ 34
*20. Macaroni Chicken* _____ 34
*21. Broccoli & Cauliflower Primavera* _____ 35
*22. Venetian Style Pasta* _____ 36
*23. Italian Beef Pasta* _____ 37
*24. Roasted Vegetables with Pasta* _____ 38

25. Chicken Pesto Pasta _____ 39
26. Slow Cooker Sausage with Spaghetti _____ 39
27. Spiced Salmon Pesto & Pasta _____ 40
28. Chicken Marinara with Pasta _____ 41
29. Breakfast Pasta _____ 42
30. Slow Cooker Italian Breakfast Casserole _____ 43
31. Slow Cooked Spaghetti _____ 43
32. Chicken Pesto _____ 44
33. Mushroom Pasta _____ 45
34. Parmesan Italian Pasta _____ 46
35. Pomodoro Pasta _____ 47
36. Pepper-Corn Pasta Salad _____ 48
37. Linguine with Fresh Tomato Sauce _____ 49
38. Spaghetti Bolognaise _____ 49
39. Pesto Fried Pasta with Chicken _____ 50
40. Pasta with Broccoli _____ 51
41. Italian Beef Curry & Pasta _____ 52
42. Spaghetti with Marinara Sauce _____ 53
43. Pasta Salad Ala Daniella _____ 54
44. Black Olives Pasta Salad _____ 55
45. Italian Pasta Salad _____ 55
46. Confetti Spaghetti Salad _____ 56
47. Aubergine & Ricotta Pasta _____ 57
48. Cold Pasta Salad _____ 58
49. Almonds, Ricotta & Wilted Green Pizza _____ 58
50. Maple & 3-Cheese Pear Pizza _____ 59
51. Roasted Vegetable Pizza _____ 61

52. White Party Pizzette _____ 62

53. Green Salad Pizza _____ 63

54. Veggie Polenta Pizza _____ 64

55. Hula Pizza _____ 65

56. Flatbread Pizza _____ 66

57. Sassy Mediterranean Pizza _____ 67

58. Bean-Veggie Pizza _____ 68

59. Tomato Cheesy Pizza _____ 69

60. Sweet Potato Pizza _____ 70

61. Low Carb Crust Pizza _____ 71

62. Chickpea Crust Pizza _____ 72

63. Veggie Gluten-Free Mini Pizza _____ 73

64. Quinoa Pizza Bites _____ 74

65. Strawberry Arugula Pizza _____ 75

66. Mini Mexican Pizza _____ 76

67. Spicy Turkey Sausage Pizza _____ 77

68. Eggplant Parmesan Pizza _____ 77

69. Black Bean Nacho Pizza _____ 78

70. Broccoli Rabe & Chicken Pizza _____ 79

71. Tomato Butter Dip _____ 81

72. Stuffed Tomatoes _____ 81

73. Tomato Gravy _____ 82

74. Tomato & Corn Salad _____ 83

75. Tomato Bites _____ 84

76. Tomato Focaccia _____ 85

77. Watermelon Tomato Salad _____ 86

78. Tomato Egg Cups _____ 87

| | |
|---|---|
| 79. Tomato Gelato | 87 |
| 80. Tomato Sliders | 88 |
| 81. Tomato Pudding | 89 |
| 82. Tomato Consommé | 90 |
| 83. Tomato Snacks | 91 |
| 84. Tomato Blossoms | 92 |
| 85. Pomegranate Tomato Salad | 93 |
| 86. Grilled Tomato Toasts | 94 |
| 87. Oil Poached Tomatoes | 95 |
| 88. Grilled (Tomato Prosciutto) Cheese | 96 |
| 89. Tomato Vinaigrette | 97 |
| 90. Hot Tomatoes | 98 |
| 91. Salsa | 99 |
| 92. Crunchy Tomatoes | 99 |
| 93. Blue Cheese Tomato Salad | 100 |
| 94. Chunky Tomato Basil Sauce | 101 |
| 95. Tomato Bread | 102 |
| 96. Tomato Cucumber Feta Salad | 103 |
| 97. Tomato Matzo Balls | 104 |
| 98. Tomato Marmalade | 105 |
| 99. Bacon Tomato Clams | 106 |
| 100. Tomato Tarte Tatin | 107 |
| 101. Polenta Gnocchi with Tomato Sauce | 108 |
| 102. Tomato Watermelon Soup | 109 |
| 103. Tomato Terrine | 110 |
| **BONUS: 27 SURPRISE RECIPES FOR SOMETHING DIFFERENT!** | 111 |

| | |
|---|---|
| 104. Taco Shells | 111 |
| 105. Taco with Wild Rice Filling | 112 |
| 106. Shrimp Taco | 113 |
| 107. Chicken Tacos | 114 |
| 108. Bacon Tacos | 115 |
| 109. Spicy Ground Turkey Taco | 116 |
| 110. Tacos with Black Beans | 117 |
| 111. Pinto Beans Taco | 118 |
| 112. Taco with Potato | 119 |
| 113. Steamed Chicken Tacos | 120 |
| 114. Tofu Tacos | 121 |
| 115. Taco with Roasted Vegetables | 122 |
| 116. Meat Ball Taco | 123 |
| 117. Egg Taco | 124 |
| 118. Baked Cauliflower Tacos | 125 |
| 119. Roasted Mushrooms Tacos | 126 |
| 120. Taco with Stir Fry Vegetables | 127 |
| 121. Taco with Mexican Salsa | 128 |
| 122. Minced Chicken Tacos | 129 |
| 123. Stir Fry Shrimp Taco | 130 |
| 124. Stir Fry Chicken Taco | 131 |
| 125. Roasted Chicken Tacos | 132 |
| 126. Wild Mushroom Taco | 133 |
| 127. Minced Beef Tacos | 134 |
| 128. Taco with Green Filling | 135 |
| 129. Egg Potato Taco | 136 |
| 130. Corn Chicken Tacos | 137 |

*Final Words* _____ *138*
*Disclaimer* _____ *140*

# Introduction

In this cookbook, you will learn how to prepare a huge array of various Italian meals. In fact, there is a focus on three particular types of recipes, pizzas, pastas and tomato-focused meals. If you feel like you need to spice up your cooking... If you feel like your family might be looking to eat something new for dinner... Or if you just enjoy cooking and want to try some new recipes... **THIS BOOK IS FOR YOU!** Enjoy!

## 1. Pizza Margherita

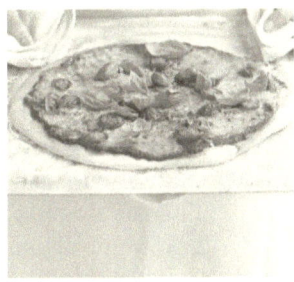

Pizza Margherita is believed to be one of the most delicious pizzas that people love.

Health-wise, it contains a good balance of fat, protein and carbohydrates. It has 360 calories per serving (two slices), 150 calories is from fat, which is a total fat of 17g, 100mg of cholesterol, 720mg of sodium, 16g of protein, 47g of carbohydrates, 400IU of Vitamin A, 3.6 mg of vitamin C, 80mg of calcium and 2.7mg of iron. These are based on a serving size of two slices.

**Ingredients**

- 1 & ¼ cup of boiling water ranging from 100º to 110º Celsius
- 3 cups and 2 tablespoons of bread flour
- 2 ½ table spoons of dry yeast
- 1 ½ table spoons of yellow cornmeal
- 5 teaspoons of olive oil
- 1 teaspoon of salt
- Cooking spray
- ½ small cups of fresh basil leaves
- 1 cup of basic pizza sauce
- 1 ½ cups of sliced mozzarella cheese
- 1 table spoon of cornmeal

**Method**

1. Put 1 cup of the boiling water in a bowl that has a stand mixer and an attachment of a dough hook. Add the flour (all 3 cups and 2 tablespoons) to the 1 cup of water and mix the two thoroughly then cover it using a plastic wrapper for 20 minutes. Add the yeast and mix it in the ¼ cup of water that remained. Allow the mixture to stay until bubbles form. Add 1/2 teaspoon of salt into the yeast mixture.

2. Add oil into the dough from step 2 and mix it thoroughly until soft. Combine both the yeast mixture and the dough. Put the combined mixture in a bowl that has a cooking spray coating and cover the surface of the dough with a little cooking spray too. Put the bowl with the dough in the refrigerator for 24 hours.

3. Get the dough out of the refrigerator and allow it to sit for about 1 hour still covered until it slowly adjusts to room temperature. Pour the dough on a baking sheet that has flour spread on it and press the dough so it's flat and spreads about 12 inches wide (thickness should be no more than half an inch). Spread some cornmeal on it.

4. Press the edges too to form a border that is nearly ½ inch thick and then cover the dough with some plastic (like a Gladwrap product). Put an oven rack at it lower position and place baking stone on the lower rack. First, heat the oven for 550⁰ Fahrenheit and heat the baking stone too. Take the plastic material off the dough and spread ¼ tablespoon of salt on it.

5. Leaving a ½ inch border, distribute the pizza sauce all over the dough and place cheese over the pizza. Move the pizza slowly onto the already heated baking stone or oven with the use of a spatula or something similar. Bake for about 11 to 12 minutes at a temperature of 550⁰. The pizza should turn golden in color. Cut the pizza dividing it into 10 wedges and spread basil on it.

**Tips and Fun Fact about Pizza Margherita**

*Queen Margherita of Italy liked eating Pizza hence the name Pizza Margherita.*

*Pizza Margherita has spread worldwide especially with it being prepared in both homes and at restaurants. This type of pizza was highly appreciated as mozzarella cheese is believed to help in the prevention of colon cancer.*

## 2. Spicy Sausage & Mushroom Pizza

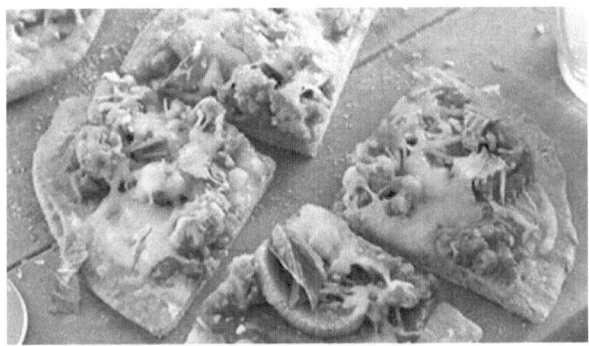

This type of pizza is commonly known as one of the healthier options because it contains a decent serving of mushrooms – which are both high in protein and also essential amino acids.

**Ingredients**

- 1 pound of fresh pizza dough
- 1 cup of sliced onions
- Cooking spray
- 5 ounces of hot Italian sausage
- 1 cup of thinly sliced onions
- 1 packet of sliced mushrooms
- 1 cup of diced green or red pepper
- 2 table spoon of yellow corn meal
- ¾ cup of sodium marinara sauce
- ¾ cup of shredded mozzarella cheese
- ½ cup of Parmigiano-Reggiano cheese

**Method**

1. First, heat the oven to temperatures of 450° Fahrenheit. Put the already mixed dough in a bowl that has a cooking spray coating. Cover the dough with a plastic wrapper and allow it stay for 15 minutes.

2. Using medium-high heat, begin heating a non-stick skillet. Apply a coating of cooking spray on the pan. Put chopped sausage pieces on the pan and cook as you stir for 3 to 4 minutes. To it, add onions and then add mushrooms and allow them to sauté for about four minutes after which you will add bell pepper and then sauté for 2 to 3 minutes.

3. Roll your dough into a 12-inch-wide circle and put it on a baking sheet that has some cornmeal on it. With an inch border being left around (for the crust), put sauce on the dough. Put the sautéed sausages on top of the dough and spread cheese on top of the sausages. Using temperatures of 450º Fahrenheit, bake it until it turns golden brown. It should take between 15-20 minutes.

**Things to Know**

*As already mentioned, mushrooms are very healthy and can provide a great balance of both proteins and other nutritional benefits.*

*Pecorino Romano is always cheaper and can substitute Parmigiano-Reggiano when making this type of pizza!*

### 3. Bacon, Tomato & Arugula Pizza

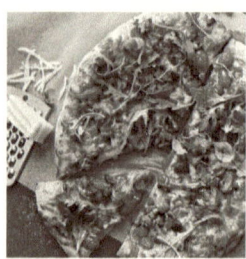

If you are in a hurry, you can make this pizza faster by warming the dough in the microwave at a slightly higher heat.

**Ingredients**

- 1 ½ cup of water
- Cooking spray
- 2 small cups of halved grape tomatoes
- 1 pound of pizza dough
- 5 apple wood-smoked bacon slices
- ½ teaspoon of crushed pepper
- 1 table spoon of yellow corn meal
- ¾ cup of marinara sauce
- 1 cup of shredded mozzarella cheese
- 1 ½ cup of baby arugula
- 1¼ teaspoons of virgin olive oil
- ¾ of white vinegar

**Method**

1. Put 1 cup of water in a bowl. Add the flour and mix until soft. And allow it to settle for about 5 minutes. Get ¼ cup of water and mix with yeast in a separate bowl. Add ¼ teaspoon of salt to this, then add the entire mixture to the dough and mix it thoroughly until soft. Cover it with a plastic wrapper and refrigerate the dough for 24 hours.

2. Please note the above step is only required if you don't already have the dough pre-made. Heat the oven at a temperature of 450° Fahrenheit. Coat a bowl with cooking spray and put the dough in the same bowl and allow it to stand for about 15 minutes while covered.

3. Take the bacon and cook it on a skillet using medium heat until it turns crisp. Take the bacon off the skillet and crumble it. After this, place it back on the pan. Then add tomatoes and pepper to the mixture in the pan. Cook for 2 to 3 minutes as you continuously stir.

4. Get the dough and roll it on a baking sheet that is sprinkled with cornmeal. Press it into a circle. Then place the sauce on top of the dough and spread, as you leave a ½ inch border. Put the tomatoes, peppers and bacon on top of it and spread cheese on top of all of it. Bake it with temperatures of 450° on an oven rack at the bottom for about 17 minutes. Serve with a mix of arugula and any other ingredients you might like on top of the pizza.

### 4. Chicken & Herb White Pizza

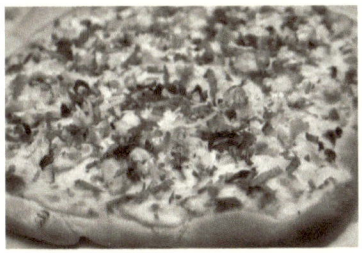

This is a great pizza to try as a change to regular ones – mainly because of the chicken!

**Ingredients**

- 1 ¼ cup of warm water
- ¼ teaspoon of salt

- 1 pound of fresh pizza dough
- Cooking spray
- 1 tablespoon butter
- 2 minced garlic cloves
- 2 tablespoons of flour
- ¾ cup of milk
- ¾ cup of pecorino Romano cheese (grated)
- 1 table spoon of yellow corn meal
- 2 cups of shredded boneless chicken
- ¼ diced red onion
- ¾ table spoon of chopped oregano
- ¾ table spoon of chopped chives
- ¾ table spoon of chopped parsley

**Method**

1. Put 1 cup of warm water in a bowl. Add the flour and mix until soft. Put ¼ cup of warm water in a bowl and add yeast and ¼ cup of salt. Stir the mixture and allow it to stay for some time until it bubbles form.

2. Put the yeast mixture into the dough and thoroughly mix. Cover the dough with a clean plastic wrapper and put it in the refrigerator for 24 hours. The above step is only required if you don't already have pre-made dough.

3. Get the dough out of the refrigerator and allow it stand for it be at room temperature. Heat the oven for about 450º Celsius. Put the dough in a bowl that has a cooking spray coating and allow it to stay for 15 minutes.

4. Put butter on a saucepan and heat partially. Put some garlic to the melted butter and stir continuously while you cook it for about 30 to 35 seconds. Add flour, then pepper to it and allow it cook for 1 minute as you stir. Turn off the heat, add cheese and stir again until the cheeses melts.

5. On the baking sheet, sprinkle cornmeal then roll the dough onto it with a thickness of no more than ½ inch. Add chicken and onions on top. Bake it at temperatures of 450º on a rack at the bottom until it turns golden brown. Let the baking take about 15-20 minutes, but keep an eye on it.

## 5. Four-Cheese Pizza

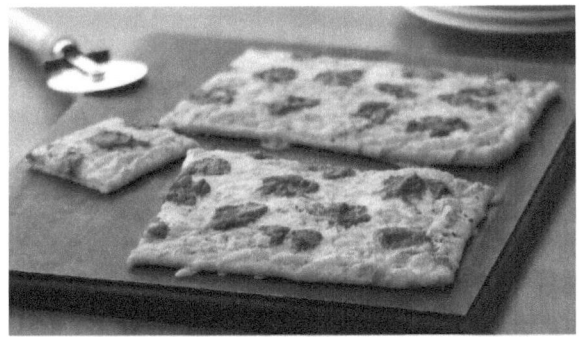

The four-cheese Pizza is a very delicious pizza that contains ricotta cheese, which has an amazing texture appearing creamy in nature and has a nice flavor. Therefore, the recipe has been voted, among the many recipes, as one of the most appetizing ones.

**Ingredients**

- 2 cups of warm water
- 2 cups and 2 tablespoons of bread flour
- 2 ¼ teaspoons of dry yeast
- 8 teaspoons of divided olive oil
- Cooking spray
- ¾ teaspoon of salt
- 1 ½ table spoons of olive oil
- 1 ¼ table spoon of yellow corn meal
- 2 table spoons of chopped garlic
- 2 ¼ of chopped fresh chives
- ¼ cup of crushed Parmigiano-Reggiano cheese
- ½ cup of crumbled Gorgonzola cheese
- 1 ¼ of sliced taleggio
- 1/3 cup of part-skim ricotta cheese

**Method**

1. Put 1 cup of warm water in a bowl that has a stand mixer. Add the flour into bowl and mix it thoroughly. Add yeast to the remaining ¼ cup of water in a bowl and mix. Let it stay for some minutes until bubbles form. Put 5 teaspoons of oil, the yeast mixture and salt into the bowl containing the dough and mix it all until soft.

2. Take a bowl, coat it with cooking spray and place the dough there and cover it. Put the dough in the refrigerator for 24 hours. Get the dough out of the refrigerator and allow it to stand for some time or it come room temperature. Roll the dough on a baking sheet containing some flour on it.

3. Press it to form a 12-inch circle. The baking sheet should be spread with cornmeal. The edges should be crimpled to form a ½ inch border, then cover the dough with a plastic material. Place the oven rack at the lowest point. Put a pizza stone on the rack at the lower point. Heat the oven up to $550^0$ and the stone for 30 minutes just before the dough is baked.

4. Take the plastic wrap away from the dough. Mix garlic and a table spoon of oil then brush the mixture over the dough as you leave a ½ inch border. Place the ricotta on the dough. Place Gorgonzola and taleggio on top of ricotta. On top of it all, place Parmigiano-Reggiano.

5. Gently move pizza onto the already heat pizza stone by use of a spatula. Bake at temperatures of $550^0$ for about 12 minutes until the color turns golden. Cut the pizza into 10 different wedges then spread chives on them.

**Fun Fact**

*The Four-cheese Pizza is believed to be tasty and healthy because it contains a balanced amount of both protein and calcium.*

*It is known as the world's best "cheesiest" pizza.*

# Read This FIRST - 100% FREE BONUS

**FOR A LIMITED TIME ONLY** – Get Olivia's best-selling book *"The #1 Cookbook: Over 170+ of the Most Popular Recipes Across 7 Different Cuisines!"* absolutely FREE!

Readers have absolutely loved this book because of the wide variety of recipes. It is highly recommended you check these recipes out and see what you can add to your home menu!

Once again, as a big thank-you for downloading this book, I'd like to offer it to you *100% FREE for a LIMITED TIME ONLY!*

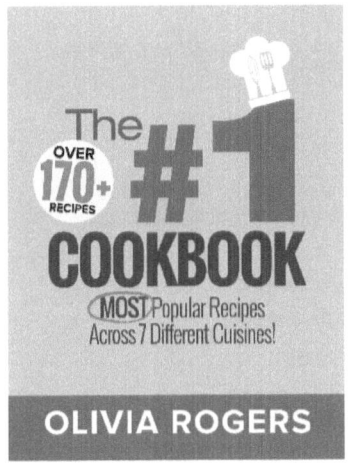

## Get your free copy at:

## TheMenuAtHome.com/Bonus

## 6. Garlicky Clam Grilled Pizza

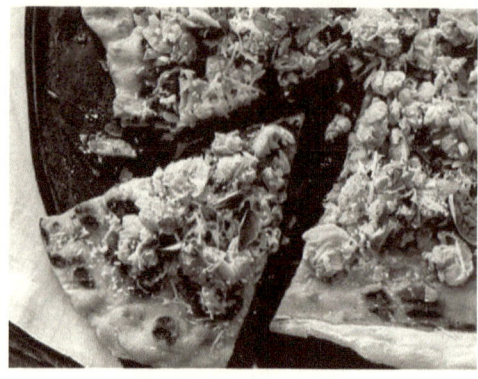

Garlicky Clam Grilled Pizza is the best choice for many who love pizzas. It is healthy and because of its slightly lower sugar content, it can be a great choice for diabetics.

**Ingredients**

- 1 ¼ cup of hot water of 100º to 110º
- 3 cups and two table spoons of bread flour
- 2 ¼ tablespoon of dry yeast
- 12 teaspoons of divided olive oil
- ½ teaspoon of salt
- Cooking spray
- 3 table spoons of yellow corn meal
- 2 tablespoons of butter
- 1/4 cup of chopped shallots
- 6 minced garlic cloves
- ¾ cup dry white wine
- 5 pack of small scrubbed clams
- 1/2 cup of crushed Parmigiano-Reggiano cheese
- 1 ½ tablespoon of chopped fresh flat-leaf parsley
- 1 tablespoon of chopped fresh oregano

**Method**

1. Put 1 cup of water in a bowl of a stand mixer. Mix flour with the 1 cup of water and mix them until they combine. Cover the mixture and let it stand for about 20 minutes. Mix ¼ of water with yeast mix and allow it to settle until bubbles appear.

2. Take salt, the yeast mixture and 5 teaspoons of oil and add them to the flour mixture and mix them put the dough in a bowl that has a cooking spray coating then cover it with a plastic material that is also coated with cooking spray. Keep the dough in a refrigerator for a whole day.

3. Get the dough from the refrigerator and let it stand until it comes to room temperature. Roll the dough and press it into a 12-inch circle on a baking sheet containing a little flour and cornmeal on it. Wrap the dough. Heat your grill up. Place a Dutch in the oven over medium heat and the add 3 tablespoons of oil to the pan and let it spread all over the pan.

4. To the pan, add butter then swirl it to allow it to melt. Add the shallots to the pan and let it sauté for 2 to three minutes. Add garlic, then let it sauté for a minute. Stir in the clams and wine and allow it to heat up. Cook it for 8 minutes while covered until you see the shells opening. Discard any shells that are not opened. Get clams out of the pan by using a spoon.

5. Pass cooking liquid through a very fine sieve allowing it to settle on the bowl, leaving behind the solid particles. Get the clams out of shells and discard the shells. Gently chop the clams and toss with reserved solids. Put the pizza dough on a grill rack that has a cooking spray coating and cornmeal on the side. Let it grill for about 4 to 5 minutes until it appears blistered.

6. Turn the dough over and grill it for some 3 minutes and then remove it out of the grill. Add the clam mixture on the top of the crust's and leave a border of ½ inch. Add cheese on the top. Get the pizza back to the grill rack and grill it for about 5 minutes to allow a thorough cooking. Add oregano and parley onto it. Cut the pizza into 5 rectangles, then 10 wedges from the rectangles.

## Fun Fact

*Garlic Clam Grilled Pizza is gaining popularity everywhere as it is easy to prepare and has a lot of nutritional benefits.*

*It is great for sea food lovers around the world.*

## 7. Smoked Salmon Thin-Crust Pizza

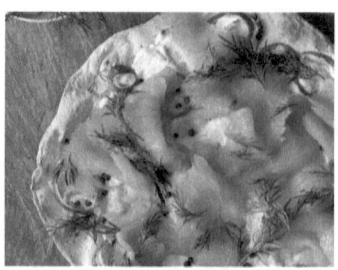

This pizza is yet another great, healthy option for pizza-lovers. The salmon is not only high in protein, but also rich in healthy fats. It also has vitamin D, and the fatty acids with high omega 3 content helps in prevention of many chronic diseases including cardiovascular diseases.

**Ingredients**

- ¾ cup of warm water
- ¾ teaspoon of dry yeast
- 2 ½ table spoons of olive oil
- ¼ teaspoon of salt
- 2 cups of bread flour
- Cooking spray
- 2 table spoons of yellow cornmeal
- ½ cup of cream cheese
- 1 ½ tablespoons of drained capers
- 5 sliced red onions
- 4 thinly sliced cold smoked salmon
- 1 ½ tablespoons of chopped fresh drill

**Method**

1. Mix ¾ cup of warm water with flour in a bowl that has a stand mixer with a dough hook attached. Allow it to stand for about 5 minutes until bubbles form. Mix water, salt and yeast and add it to the mixture. Mix the whole thing until soft. Coat a large bowl with cooking spray and place the dough in and cover it with some plastic wrapping.

2. Place the bowl with the dough in the refrigerator. Place the oven rack at the lowest position. Put a pizza stone on the lowest rack too. First, heat the oven to a temperature of $550^0$. Heat the pizza stone before you bake the dough for about 30 minutes. Get the dough out of the refrigerator, remove the plastic wrapper and allow it to stand until it returns to room temperature.

3. Roll the dough to a thin, 13-inch-wide circle on top of a baking sheet containing some flour and sprinkled with cornmeal. Crimp the edges and make sure it forms a ½ inch border. Using a fork, pierce the dough a few times.

4. Move the dough slowly over the preheated pizza stone by use of a spatula. Bake at a temperature of 550⁰ for 4 to 5 minutes. Remove it from the oven and place the cheese all over the dough. Spread onions and some capers round the cheese. Bake it for about 5 minutes until it is golden brown. Add the salmon on top. Cut the pizza into wedges.

**Fun Fact**

*Beside this pizza tasting great, the salmon also helps reduce inflammation, is said to improve vision, helps with cancer prevention, aids skin and hair health and assists in solving cognitive problems.*

*Why not try this pizza for dinner tomorrow?*

## 8. Pepperoni Deep-Dish Pizza

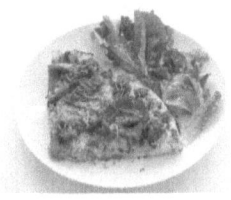

**Ingredients**

- 1 ½ cup of hot water
- 3 cups of bread flour
- 5 teaspoons of olive oil
- ¾ teaspoons of salt
- Cooking spray
- 1 ½ cups of shredded mozzarella cheese
- 1 ¾ of basic pizza source
- 2 ¼ ounces of pepperoni slices
- 2 ¼ tablespoons of crushed Parmigiano-Reggiano cheese

**Method**

1. Put 1 cup of hot water in a bowl that has a stand mixer. Pour the flour into the water in the bowl and mix thoroughly. Add yeast to the

remaining ¼ cup of water in another bowl and mix. Let it sit for about five minutes until bubbles form. Put 5 teaspoons of oil, the yeast mixture and salt into the bowl containing the dough and mix it until soft.

2. Take a bowl, coat it with cooking spray and place the dough there and cover it well with plastic wrapping. Put the dough in the refrigerator for a day. Get the dough out of the refrigerator and allow it to sit for some time until it adjusts to room temperature. Flatten the dough and then place it in a baking tray that has been coated with some cooking spray.

3. In your oven, on a bottom rack, place a baking sheet and heat the oven at temperatures of $450^0$. Place ¾ cup of mozzarella on the pizza dough. Add pepperoni, pizza sauce, Parmigiano-Reggiano, and a ½ cup of mozzarella. Put it in the oven and bake for about 25 minutes at $450^0$ until the crust turns golden brown. Cut the pizza into 6 rectangles.

**Fun Fact**

*The name pepperoni is derived from pepper, which refers to the spicy peppers added in the preparation of it.*

*Unlike any other type of pizza, the Pepperoni deep-dish pizza is loved by many, especially during parties. It is one of America's favorite pizza.*

## 9. Veggie Grilled Pizza

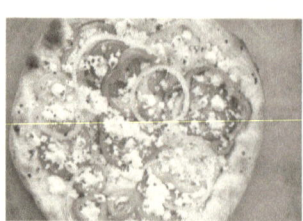

Just as the name describes, the Veggie Grilled Pizza has a high content of vegetable, therefore is very healthy type of pizza.

Vegetables, as I'm sure you probably already know, are great to eat everyday due to their various vitamins and minerals. They are also fantastic sources of antioxidants. They also have soluble and insoluble dietary fiber too, which helps with digestion.

**Ingredients**

- 1 ½ cups of water
- 3 cups of bread flour
- 2 ½ teaspoons of dry yeast
- 12 teaspoons of olive oil
- 1 ¼ teaspoons of salt
- Cooking spray
- 3 table spoons of yellow cornmeal
- 13 ounces of sliced baby eggplant
- 1 ½ of thick sliced medium zucchini
- 1 ½ red bell paper
- 4 minced garlic cloves
- ¾ basic pizza sauces
- 1 ½ cups of shredded fontina cheese
- ½ cups of small mint leaves
- 2 ½ teaspoons of fresh thyme leaves

**Method**

1. Put 1 cup of warm water in a bowl that has a stand mixer. Add the flour into the water in the bowl and mix it thoroughly. Mix yeast with the remaining ¼ cup of water in another bowl. Let the mixture sit for a few minutes until bubbles form. Put 5 teaspoons of oil, the yeast mixture and salt into the bowl containing the dough and mix it until soft. Take a bowl, coat it with cooking spray and place the dough inside. Wrap the dough well with plastic wrapping and put it in the refrigerator for a day.

2. The next day, prepare the grill to dry high. Get the dough out of the refrigerator and allow it to sit for some time or until it adjusts to room temperature. Take the dough and flatten it into a 12-inch circle on a baking sheet that is lightly floured and spread with cornmeal. Let the edge form a ½ inch border by crimping it and then slightly cover the dough with a plastic wrapper.

3. Take 2 tablespoons of oil and brush it on the eggplant and on the bell pepper. Brush it on the zucchini too. Grill the eggplant for about 4 minutes on both sides to make it soft then put it in a bowl. Grill the zucchini for 3 to 4 minutes on each side then add to the eggplant.

4. Take a zip top plastic bag and put the pepper in it, seal it and let it sit in there for less than 10 minutes. Then take it out and add peeled pepper to the mixture containing the vegetables. Chop the vegetables in larger

sizes and then add garlic to the vegetables and toss to combine. Put the pizza dough with cornmeal on the upper side, on the grill rack that has a cooking spray coating, then grill it for 4 to 5 minutes until it blisters.

5. Turn the dough over and grill for 3 minutes then remove from grill. Place pizza sauce over the top of the crust leaving a ½ inch border. Put the vegetable mixture evenly over the sauce and sprinkle randomly with a ½ teaspoon of salt together with black pepper. Add cheese on the top and return the pizza to the grill rack, grilling it for about 4 minutes until it is cooked thoroughly. Cut the pizza into 10 pieces and sprinkle mint and thyme on it.

### 10. Quick Pizza Margherita

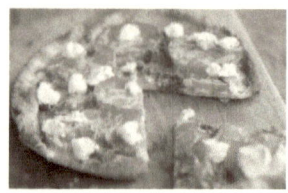

The Quick Pizza Margherita is believed to be first introduced in Italy, therefore cooked and eaten by many Italians. It is a delicious type of pizza that is cheaper than any other and as usual, it can be easily cooked.

**Ingredients**

- 2 ½ cups of pizza crust dough
- Cooking spray
- 1 ½ teaspoons of extra virgin oil
- 1 ½ halved garlic cloves
- 6 thinly sliced plum tomatoes
- 1 ½ cup of shredded mozzarella cheese
- 1 ½ teaspoon of balsamic vinegar
- ¾ of sliced fresh basil
- 1/8 teaspoon of salt
- 1/8 teaspoon of fresh black pepper

**Method**

1. Preheat oven at temperatures of 400º. Take the dough and unroll it onto a baking sheet that is coated with cooking spray. Cut it into a rectangular form of 13x11 inches. Bake at a temperature of 400º for, at most, 9 minutes.

2. Get the crust out of the oven and slowly rub a ½ teaspoon of oil over it. Use garlic to rub the crust too. Place tomatoes slices on the crust creating a ½ inch border between. Sprinkle cheese all over. Bake for about 12 minutes at temperatures of 400°. Allow the cheese to melt and the crust to turn golden.

3. Mix a ½ teaspoon of oil with vinegar and stir thoroughly. Evenly spread pizza together with sliced basil, pepper and salt. Sprinkle the vinegar mixture evenly along the pizza and then cut the pizza into 8 pieces.

## 11. Greek Lamb Pizza

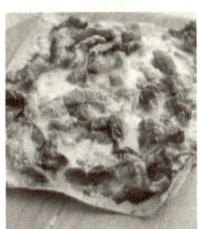

**Ingredients**

- 1 Italian cheese thin pizza crust
- 1 cup of marinara sauce
- 3 serving lamb steaks and grilled onions
- ¾ cups of crumbled feta cheese
- ½ cups of mozzarella cheese
- ¼ cup of sliced pepperoncini pepper

**Method**

1. Preheat the oven at 450°. Put the pizza crust on a baking sheet. Spread the marinara sauce over the crust as you leave a ½ inch border. Evenly spread lamb steaks together with Herbes de Provence and grilled sweet onions. Sprinkle it with feta mozzarella cheeses.

2. Bake the pizza for about 12 minutes at temperatures of 450° until the cheeses melt. Get the pizza from the oven and sprinkle it with pepperoncini peppers. Cut the pizza into 8 wedges.

## 12. Arugula Pizza with Poached Eggs

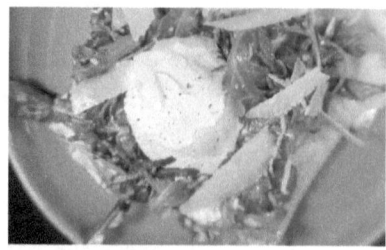

Arugula, one of the vegetable contents found in this pizza, is originally from the Mediterranean. It is also known as fresh salad rocket.

The biggest health benefit is how low in calories it is. Also, the leaves contain both iron and copper. Besides that, it has high levels of vitamins K, C and A plus many other beneficial nutrients.

**Ingredients**

- Cooking spray
- ¾ cup of shaved Romano cheese
- 1 pack of refrigerated pizza crust
- 1 ½ tablespoon of white vinegar
- 8 eggs
- 1 package of baby arugula
- 5 teaspoons of virgin olive oil
- ¾ of grated fresh lemon rind
- 1 ½ tablespoon of lemon juice
- 1/8 teaspoon of salt
- ¼ teaspoon of fresh black pepper

**Methods**

1. Preheat the oven at 450⁰. Take your pizza dough and unroll it on a baking sheet that has a slight coating of cooking spray. Bake continuously as oven heats for about seven minutes. Mix the ¼ cup of Romano with ricotta and remove it from pan oven. Spread cheese mixture as fast as possible over the dough as you leave a ½ inch border on the edges. Put the pan back to the oven and bake for about 5 minutes.

2. As the pizza is baking, add 2/3 cup of water to the large skillet and let it boil. Reduce heat and allow it to simmer. Add vinegar, then break each of the eggs into a custard cup and pour into the pan. Cook for about three minutes then remove the pan by use of a slotted spoon.

3. Mix the ¼ cup of Romano cheese that remained with arugula and the four ingredients plus salt in a bowl. Place the arugula mixture and eggs on top of pizza. Sprinkle a bit of pepper on the pizza and cut into 6 pieces.

**Fun Facts**

*Arugula contains folate which is a good source of folic acid.*

## 13. Peach & Gorgonzola Chicken Pizza

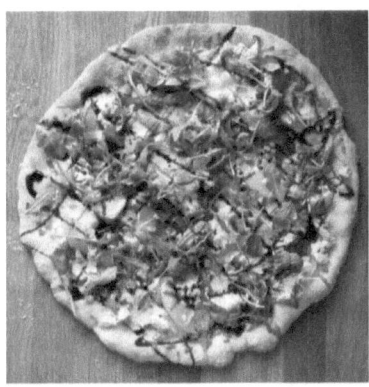

Gorgonzola on pizza is an Italian blue cheese that is found all over Italy. It's high in calcium, potassium and protein, which makes the Peach & Gorgonzola Chicken Pizza a great choice for you.

Peach is also in this pizza and it is low in calories and has no saturated fat.

**Ingredients**

- 2 backed pizza crust
- Cooking spray
- 1½ teaspoons of extra virgin olive oil
- ¾ cup of mozzarella cheese
- 1 ½ cups of shredded cooked chicken
- ½ cups of crumbled Gorgonzola cheese
- 1 thinly sliced unpeeled peach
- ½ cup of balsamic vinegar

**Method**

1. Heat the oven first, for about 400°. Put the pizza crust on a baking sheet that has a cooking spray coating and gently brush 1 teaspoon of extra virgin oil all over the crust.

2. Add ¼ cup of shredded mozzarella cheese, peach, gorgonzola cheese, and then the chicken. Bake for about 11 minutes at 400° until it turns golden brown. Cut it into 8 wedges.

**Fun Fact**

*This pizza can help you deal with any constipation (if you are having problems with this) due to the high levels of potassium. Also, this is a cheap pizza to make for the whole family!*

## 14. Roasted Vegetable & Ricotta Pizza

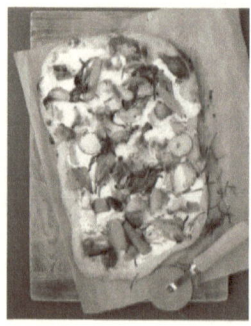

Roasted vegetable and ricotta pizza is highly nutritional especially with the mushroom, since it contains essential amino acids and is high in protein. Preparing such a pizza is quite simple and can be done by anybody.

**Ingredients**

- 1 ½ pounds of fresh pizza dough
- 2 ½ cups of sliced mushrooms
- 1 cup of sliced zucchini
- ¼ teaspoon of fresh black pepper
- 1 ½ yellow fresh, sliced bell pepper
- 1 ½ thick-sliced red onion
- 6 teaspoons of olive oil
- 1 ¼ tablespoons of yellow cornmeal
- ½ cup of tomato sauce
- 1 ¼ cups of mozzarella cheese
- ½ teaspoons of fresh crushed red pepper

- ½ cup of part-skim ricotta cheese
- 2 table spoons of basil leaves

**Method**

1. Heat oven at about 200ºC. Put two large baking trays in the oven and heat them for 10 minutes. Gently put 1 tablespoon of tomato sauce over each pizza. Sprinkle the chargrill pan or barbecue plate with a bit of oil and place over medium heat. Grill capsicum, eggplant, squash and zucchini for about 4 minutes to make it tender.

2. Place grilled vegies over prepared base in layers. Place drops of pesto and ricotta on top then sprinkle a bit mozzarella on it. Transfer the pizzas onto different trays. Bake them for about 14 minutes until they appear brownish. Add rocket leaves on top. Cut into wedges of your size choice and serve.

### 15. Artichoke & Arugula Pizza with Prosciutto

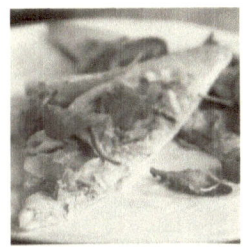

The Artichoke & Arugula Pizza with Prosciutto is a great pizza if you enjoy variations – and best of all is that it will help with digestion as well as have a slight detoxing effect.

**Ingredients**

- Cooking spray
- 1 ½ tablespoon of cornmeal
- 1 can of pizza crust dough
- 3 table spoons of commercial presto
- ¾ cup of shredded part-skim mozzarella cheese
- 1 ½ package of thawed and drained frozen artichoke
- 1 ½ ounces of sliced prosciutto
- 3 tablespoons of parmesan cheese (shredded)
- 2 cups of arugula leaves
- ¾ tablespoons of fresh lemon juice

**Method**

1. Put the oven rack at its lowest position and preheat it at 500°. Roll your dough on a baking sheet that is coated with cooking spray and cornmeal. Part the dough into a rectangle of approximately 14x10 inches. Carefully spread the presto on the dough leaving borders of ½ inches. Add mozzarella cheese on top of presto.

2. Place a baking sheet on the oven rack at the bottom and bake for 5 minutes at 500° then remove the pizza from oven. Chop the artichokes and arrange them on the pizza. On the top, place sliced prosciutto. Sprinkle some parmesan on it.

3. Put the pizza back into the oven and bake for 6 minutes more until brown in color. Put arugula in a bowl and drizzle some juice over the arugula. Add the arugula mixture on top of the pizza. Cut the pizza into small rectangles of about 7x5 inches then cut the rectangles into wedges.

### 16. Supreme Pizza

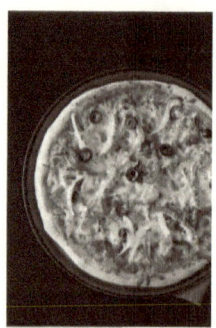

Supreme pizza is a slightly higher calorie pizza; however, the flavors are amazing. This is definitely one that you may want to eat in moderation.

**Ingredients**

- 1 ½ of fresh pizza crushed dough
- Cooking spray
- 2 ½ teaspoons of olive oil
- 2 turkey Italian sausage link
- 1 ½ cups of sliced mushrooms
- 1 cup of fresh sliced red bell pepper

- 1 cup of fresh sliced orange bell pepper
- 1 ½ cup of thinly sliced red onions
- 1/4 teaspoon of crushed red pepper
- 3 of sliced garlic cloves
- 3/4 cup of lower-sodium marinara sauce
- 5 ounces of thinly sliced mozzarella cheese

**Method**

1. Place the oven rack at its lowest position and preheat it at 500º. Put the dough on a baking sheet that has a cooking spray coating and sprinkled lightly with flour. Roll the dough into a 14-inch circle. Place the circle on a 14-inch pizza pan coated with cooking spray.

2. Place the large nonstick skillet on heat then place some oil on it and let it heat a bit. Add sausage to the pan and cook for 2 to 3 minutes as you stir to make them crumble. Add bell pepper, mushrooms, red crushed pepper, onion and garlic and let the mixture sauté for 4 minutes as you stir continuously.

3. Place the sauce all over the dough leaving a border of less than 2 inches. Place the cheese on top of the sauce. Arrange the turkey mixture randomly over the cheese. Bake for about 15 minutes at 500º till cheese and crust turns brown. Cut it into 6 rectangles then cut the rectangles to come up with 12 wedges.

### 17. Apricot & Prosciutto Thin-Crust Pizza

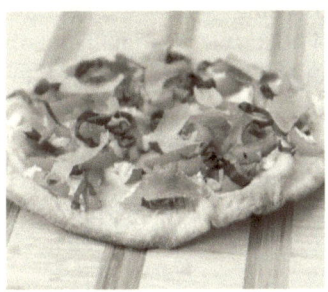

The apricots in this pizza not only provide a great hint of sweetness, but are also a rich source of anti-oxidants. It is high in fiber and great for your heart. Overall, it is a nice meal to add to your diet and easy to prepare.

**Ingredients**

- ¾ cup of warm water
- ¾ teaspoon of dry yeast
- 9 teaspoons of olive oil
- ¾ teaspoons of salt
- Bread flour
- Cooking spray
- Cornmeal
- 1 ½ teaspoons of chopped thyme
- ½ of ground black pepper
- Apricots cut into 8 wedges
- 3 peeled and thinly sliced shallots
- 1 cup of crumbled goat cheese
- 1 ¾ tablespoons of chopped flat leaf parsley
- 1 ½ tablespoons of minced fresh chives
- 1 ¼ cup of arugula
- 1 ¼ ounce of thinly sliced prosciutto
- 1 ¼ ounce of shaved Parmigiano-Reggiano cheese

**Method**

1. Put 1 cup of warm water in a bowl that has a stand mixer. Add the flour into the water in the bowl and mix it thoroughly. Add yeast to the remaining ¼ cup of water in a bowl and mix. Let it stand for about five minutes until bubbles form. Mix salt, 5 teaspoons of oil and the yeast mixture into the bowl containing the dough and mix it until soft.

2. Take a bowl, coat it with cooking spray and place the dough there. Cover the dough using a plastic material. Put the dough in the refrigerator for 24 hours. Get the dough out of the refrigerator and allow it to stand for about an hour for it to adjust to room temperature.

3. Place the dough onto a baking sheet that is lightly floured and has some cornmeal on it. Roll the dough into a 12-inch circle. The edges should form a border of about ½ inches. Make small holes in the dough by piercing it using a fork then cover it using a plastic material.

4. Place the oven rack at the lowest position then place a pizza stone on the lowest rack and heat the oven up to $550°$ and the pizza stone for about 30 minutes. Mix thyme, pepper, shallots, 1 tablespoon of oil, apricots and ¼ teaspoon of salt. Unwrap the dough and pass the dough slightly onto the already hot pizza stone by use of a spatula. Bake for 5 minutes at temperatures of $550°$.

5. Add goat cheese and apricot mixture at the top of the dough and bake for five more minutes until golden brown. Cut the pizza into 10 slices and sprinkle chive and parsley the slices. With the remaining 1 ½ teaspoons of oil, toss the arugula. Add Parmigiano-Reggiano cheese and prosciutto on top then cut into 10 wedges and serve it.

## 18. Rustic Pasta Toss

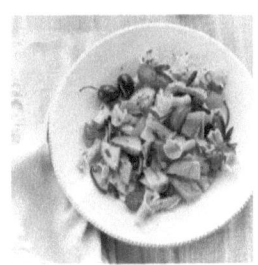

This meal is delicious and filling and will tempt you into multiple servings.

**Ingredients**

- 1-pound fusilli
- 2 medium zucchini
- 1 yellow squash
- 2 pounds tomatoes
- ¼ cup each of pitted olives and virgin olive oil
- 3 tablespoon red wine vinegar
- 2 cans tuna in water
- 1 garlic clove
- Salt and pepper

**Method**

1. Boil pasta in a large saucepan filled with water until pasta is tender but firm. Trim and cut zucchini and squash first into quarters length-wise then thin slices across. Chop tomatoes and slice the olives

2. Whisk vinegar, ¼ teaspoon salt, $^1/_8$ teaspoon ground pepper, oil and garlic then stir in the tomatoes. Add well drained pasta and tuna to tomato mixture. Add the rest of the stuff in and toss well.

**Did you know?**

*Tomato is not a vegetable but a fruit. It contains anthocyanin which helps you keep your memory sharp and fully focused.*

## 19. Italian Tilapia Parmesan with Pasta

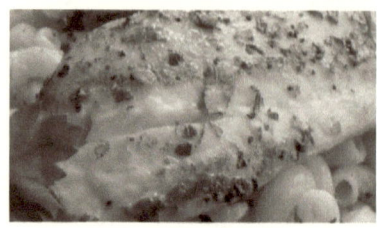

Fish has healthy fats and gives health advantages for our bodies.

## Ingredients

- 2 pounds tilapia
- 2 ounces parmesan cheese
- ¼ cup butter
- 3 tablespoons Italian dressing
- ¼ teaspoon each of garlic powder and pepper
- A small onion, chopped
- Italian seasoning
- 1-pound spaghetti

## Method

1. Spray non-stick spray at the base of the crock pot. Carefully place fish and season lightly. Mix all the other ingredients except cheese, spaghetti and dressing and spoon mixture on top of fish. Cook on low heat for three hours. Add cheese and dressing on top and cook for a further hour.

2. In the last 15 minutes, cook spaghetti according to packet instructions and drain. Place in warmed serving dishes and put individual portions on top.

## Did you know?

*Tilapia is a good source of Omega 3 fatty acids.*

## 20. Macaroni Chicken

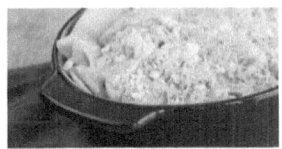

You cannot go wrong with macaroni and chicken. Both are delicious and nutritious.

**Ingredients**

- 4 ounces elbow macaroni
- 2 sliced green onions
- ½ tablespoon butter
- ½ cup halved cherry tomatoes
- 4 ounces salted chicken breast cut into small pieces
- ¼ cup halved green olives
- ½ diced red bell pepper
- 4 ounces Italian salad dressing
- Pepper

**Method**

1. Boil macaroni according to packet instructions, drain and set aside. Melt butter in a saucepan and sauté the chicken until tender. Combine everything in a large bowl and finish off with stirring in the salad dressing.

**Did you know?**

*Chicken has niacin which is essential for brain health can protect against Alzheimer's disease and dementia.*

## 21. Broccoli & Cauliflower Primavera

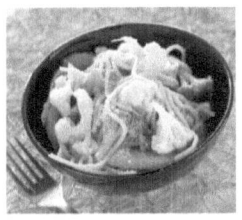

The health benefits of this dish are numerous; get healthy as you enjoy scrumptious food.

**Ingredients**

- ¼ cup olive oil
- 1-pound cauliflower florets
- 1-pound broccoli florets
- 1 pound sliced carrots
- 18 ounces screws pasta
- ½ cup grated parmesan cheese

**Method**

1. Boil pasta according to package instructions and drain. In a frying pan, heat oil and add vegetables. Season with salt and pepper. Fry for 4 minutes ensuring you don't overcook. Add pasta and mix well. Sprinkle with cheese and serve.

**Did you know?**

*Olive oil is rich in anti-oxidants which help protect the body against free radicals.*

## 22. Venetian Style Pasta

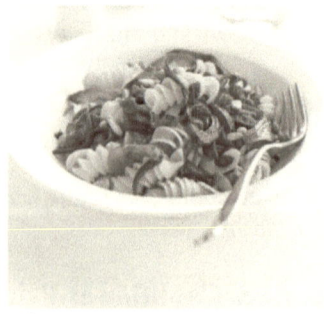

This mouth-watering dish will leave you licking the eating utensils.

**Ingredients**

- 2 sliced onions
- 1 tablespoon olive oil
- 8 ounces pasta screws
- 4 teaspoon balsamic vinegar
- 2 tablespoon each raisins and toasted pine nuts

- 5 ounces spinach, chopped

**Method**

1. Boil pasta for 8-10 minutes. Put oil in pan and fry onions till slightly brown. Stir in vinegar, raisins, capers and most of the nuts into onions and cook for 2 minutes. Stir in spinach with a little water. Toss drained pasta with mixture and divide. Scatter remaining nuts into serving dishes. Serve with roast beef.

**Did you know?**

*Olive oil is rich in the anti-oxidant hydroxytyrosol. It protects the body against free radical damage.*

### 23. Italian Beef Pasta

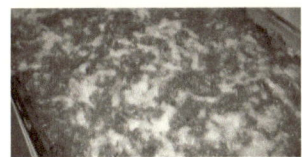

Mushrooms are healthy and beneficial for those on weight loss endeavors.

**Ingredients**

- 1-pound beef rump steak, thinly sliced across the grain into ½cm thick pieces
- 1-pound tagliatelle pasta, broken into shorter pieces
- 1 cm long chunk fresh ginger, chopped
- 12 ounces spring greens, sliced
- 6 ounces pack sliced mushrooms
- 4 tablespoon pesto sauce
- 2 tablespoon each marinara sauce and olive oil

**Method**

1. Mix sauces and set aside. Cook pasta as instructed on packet, drain and set aside. Heat a deep skillet until smoking hot, add 1 tsp oil; stir-fry meat until browned all over. Remove meat and wipe skillet.

2. Add a little more oil. Stir-fry ginger until golden. Add greens and mushrooms. Stir and cook for 3. Add steak and marinara sauce mixture.

Cook for 3 more minutes until sauce thickens a little and everything is thoroughly warmed. Place pasta in pre-warmed serving dish and top with meat dish.

**Did you know?**

*Mushrooms are among the oldest living vegetables and have been used as medicine for thousands of years.*

## 24. Roasted Vegetables with Pasta

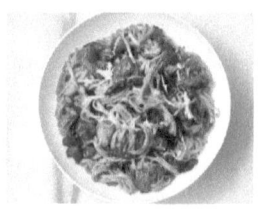

You will enjoy the flavor and yummy taste in this appetizing and filling dish.

**Ingredients**

- 8 ounces mostaccioli pasta
- 1-pound fresh mixed vegetables
- 1 teaspoon dried Italian seasoning
- 2 tablespoons each of olive oil and grated parmesan cheese
- 2 teaspoons balsamic vinegar
- ¼ cup chicken broth
- Salt and pepper

**Method**

1. Preheat oven to $220^0$ C. Boil pasta in a large pot with a lot of water until al dente, drain well. Meanwhile, slice vegetables and arrange them in a baking tray; in a single layer. Season with salt, pepper and dried seasoning and drizzle a little oil. Roast until vegetables caramelize. Mix everything and toss before serving.

**Did you know?**

*The Chinese are believed to have eaten pasta as early as 5000 B.C.*

## 25. Chicken Pesto Pasta

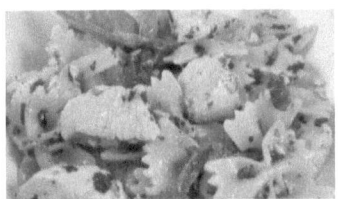

This dish is mouth-watering and scrumptious. Beware of getting second servings.

### Ingredients

- 10 skinless and boneless chicken thighs cut into strips
- 2 tablespoons olive oil
- 8 ounces cream
- Zest and juice of one lemon
- ¼ cup basil pesto
- 1-pound pasta

### Method

1. Cook pasta according to packet instructions. In the mean-time, heat oil in a wide pan and cook salted and peppered chicken for 4 minutes. Turn-over and cook for 4 more minutes then add the pesto, lemon zest and juice. Coat chicken in the pesto and stir in cream. Simmer for 4 minutes. Turn the pasta onto a serving dish and top with chicken pesto.

### Did you know?

*Chicken is niacin rich and niacin is essential for brain health.*

## 26. Slow Cooker Sausage with Spaghetti

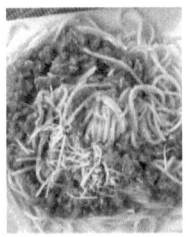

This mouth-watering dish will leave you licking the eating utensils.

**Ingredients**

- 2 pounds beef sausage
- 48 ounces spaghetti sauce
- 1 small can tomato puree
- Thinly sliced red pepper
- 1 small onion, sliced
- 1 tablespoon, cheese
- 1 cup water

**Method**

1. Cover in water and simmer sausage in skillet for ten minutes then drain. Place all the other ingredients in a crock pot. Add sausage and cook covered on low, for 3 hours. Increase heat to high and cook for an hour more. Cut sausages as desired and serve over boiled spaghetti.

**Fun fact**

*Limburger cheese and humans share a common bacterium which causes the cheese's unpleasant odor and unpleasant human odor.*

## 27. Spiced Salmon Pesto & Pasta

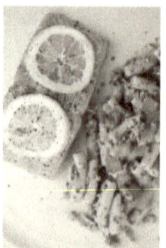

Honey gives this dish numerous health benefits including boosting immunity and helping with digestion.

**Ingredients**

- 4 x 6 ounces salmon fillets
- 2 teaspoon chili sauce
- 2 tablespoon pesto
- 1 teaspoon honey
- ¼ teaspoon each of ground red pepper and salt

- ⅛ teaspoon garlic powder
- 1-pound elbow pasta

**Method**

1. Preheat cooking spray coated broiler. Combine all ingredients except fish in a bowl and stir with a fork. Rub mixture evenly over fish. Place fillets on broiler, skin-side down. Broil for 8-10 minutes. Meanwhile, cook pasta as per packet instructions, drain and place in serving dish. Top with fish dish.

**Did you know?**

*Chili is speeds up the metabolic process and can help with weight loss.*

## 28. Chicken Marinara with Pasta

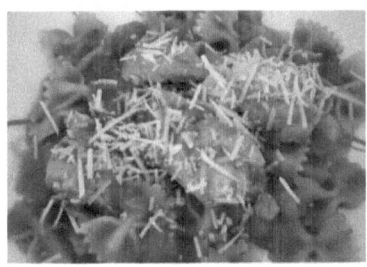

You will enjoy the flavor and yummy taste in this appetizing and filling dish.

**Ingredients**

- 1-pound fusilli pasta
- 1/2 pound of broccoli
- 1/2 pound of bacon strips
- 2 large chicken breasts
- ½ cup marinara

**Method**

1. Butter the slow cooker and put the bacon strips in layers. Add a layer of broccoli then a chicken breast. Put a second layer of bacon, followed by broccoli and then the last breast. Put last bacon layer and last broccoli layer and add 1½ cups of water.

2. Cook on low for five to six hours then mix with marinara sauce. Cook pasta as directed on packet, drain and put in serving dish. Top with chicken marinara.

**Did you know?**

*Broccoli has beneficial components found in vegetables which prevent hormone related cancers.*

### 29. Breakfast Pasta

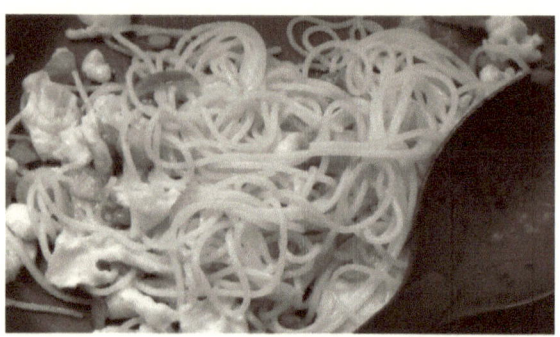

A scrumptious breakfast to keep you going for hours.

**Ingredients**

- 8 ounces rotini pasta
- 3 large eggs
- 1 tablespoon butter
- ¼ cup parmesan cheese
- 2 teaspoons pilacca

**Method**

1. Boil pasta in a large pot with a lot of water until tender but firm, drain. Melt butter in a non-stick saucepan and add pasta. Crack eggs into saucepan and scramble. Place in serving dish and add salt, hot sauce and finish by sprinkling parmesan.

**Did you know?**

*Eating cheese in moderation helps prevent tooth decay and protects enamel like most tooth pastes.*

## 30. Slow Cooker Italian Breakfast Casserole

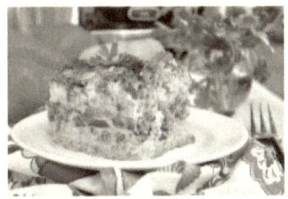

This is a filling breakfast dish that has nutrients to keep you going and filled for several hours.

**Ingredients**

- ½ pound ground Italian sausage, browned and drained
- 6 large eggs
- ½ cup milk
- 1-pound frozen hash-browns
- ½ cup pesto
- ½ cup grated parmesan cheese
- ½ pound pasta
- Salt and pepper to taste

**Method**

1. Spray non-stick cooking spray into crock pot. Thoroughly mix together beaten eggs, milk and salt and pepper before pouring into the cooker. Add remaining ingredients and stir a little. Cook on low heat for six hours until mixture sets at the center.

**Did you know?**

*Egg protein is an essential component of neurotransmitters which help communication between brain cells.*

## 31. Slow Cooked Spaghetti

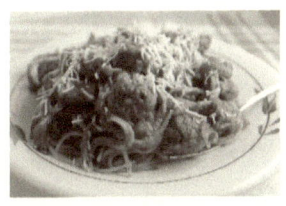

Mushrooms are healthy and very low-calorie delicacy.

**Ingredients**

- 1½ pounds minced beef
- 1½ teaspoon Italian seasoning
- 2 tablespoon dried onions
- ½ teaspoon garlic powder
- 6 ounces, cooked mushrooms
- 16 ounces tomato sauce
- 6 ounces spaghetti, broken into pieces
- Salt and pepper to taste

**Method**

1. Fry minced beef in skillet until browned. Place into slow cooker and stir in all the ingredients save for spaghetti. Cook on medium for 4 hours. Stir in spaghetti and cook on high for an additional 1 hour. Increase time if not cooked to satisfaction.

**Did you know?**

*Garlic has been used in food and medicine for more than five thousand years.*

## 32. Chicken Pesto

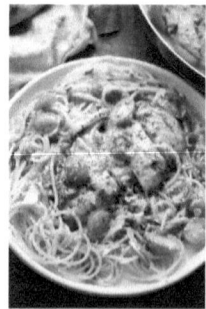

Pesto makes this dish a yummy Italian dish that you will find irresistible.

**Ingredients**

- 10 skinless and boneless chicken thighs cut into strips
- 2 tablespoons olive oil
- 8 ounces cream

- Zest and juice of one lemon
- ¼ cup basil pesto
- 1-pound pasta

**Method**

1. Cook pasta according to packet instructions. In the mean-time, heat oil in a wide pan and cook salted and peppered chicken for 4 minutes. Turn-over and cook for 4 more minutes then add pesto, lemon zest and juice. Coat chicken in pesto and stir in cream. Simmer for 4 minutes. Turn pasta onto a serving dish and top with chicken pesto.

**Did you know?**

*Chicken is niacin rich and niacin is essential for brain health.*

## 33. Mushroom Pasta

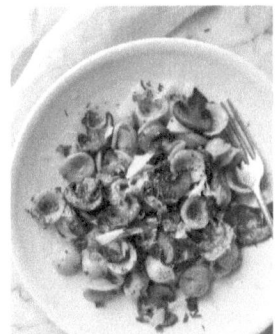

Mushrooms are healthy and beneficial for those on weight loss endeavors; they are a low-calorie delicacy.

**Ingredients**

- 1-pound linguine pasta
- 2 tablespoons butter
- 1 pound sliced mushrooms
- 3 crushed garlic cloves
- 1 cup cream
- 3 tablespoons grated parmesan cheese
- Seasoning

**Method**

1. Cook pasta as directed on packet until almost tender then drain. In a saucepan over medium heat, melt butter and cook garlic for a minute. Add mushrooms and cook covered for 10 – 15 minutes.

2. Add seasoning. Add cream, stirring frequently until thickened. Put pasta in a warmed serving dish and top with mushroom mixture. Sprinkle cheese before serving.

**Did you know?**

*Garlic has been used in food and medicine for more than five thousand years. It is also a source of selenium.*

### 34. Parmesan Italian Pasta

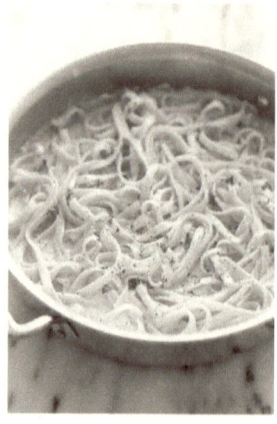

You will enjoy the flavor and yummy taste in this appetizing and filling dish.

**Ingredients**

- 1-pound elbow pasta
- 1 minced garlic clove
- 2 teaspoon capers
- 20 black olives
- 10 ounces can chopped tomatoes
- Pinch of dried oregano
- Olive oil
- Parmesan cheese

**Method**

1. Cook pasta in a pot of water until tender but firm. Meanwhile stir fry all ingredients except tomato, oregano and cheese, for a minute. Add oregano and tomato then bring mixture to the boil. Lower heat and simmer for 8 minutes, stirring at intervals. Serve with pasta and sprinkle cheese on top.

**Did you know?**

*Tomato is not a vegetable but a fruit. It contains anthocyanin which helps you keep your memory sharp and fully focused.*

### 35. Pomodoro Pasta

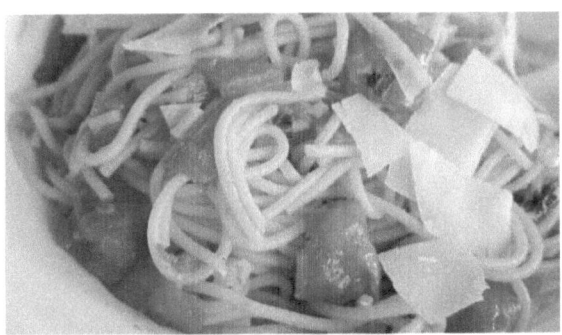

**Ingredients**

- 12 ounces ripe and de-skinned tomatoes, diced
- 12 leaves fresh basil
- 1 tablespoon olive oil
- 2 peeled and quartered cloves of garlic
- 10 ounces cooked and drained pasta

**Method**

1. Heat olive oil in saucepan and fry garlic making sure not to burn it. Add tomato and cook for 3 minutes. Add salt and pepper then add in torn basil leaves.

2. Remove and discard garlic then stir the mixture well. Combine pasta and sauce in a pre-warmed bowl and toss. Squirt olive oil and serve with grated parmesan.

**Did you know?**

*Garlic has been used in food and medicine for more than five thousand years. It is also a source of selenium.*

## 36. Pepper-Corn Pasta Salad

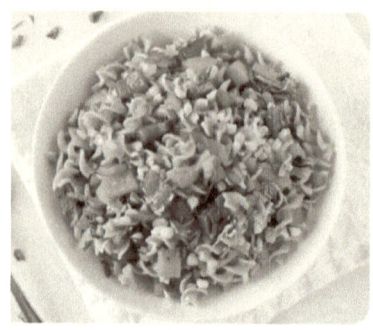

**Ingredients**

- 8 ounces pasta of choice
- 1 chopped avocado
- 1 tablespoon olive oil
- 1 chopped onion
- ¾ cup corn kennels
- 2 tablespoon fresh lime juice
- Salt and pepper to taste
- ½ cup roasted pepper, chopped

**Method**

1. Cook pasta according to packet instructions and drain. In the meantime, fry onion in a large saucepan over medium heat for 2 minutes.

2. Stir in the corn and cook for 2 more minutes before adding pepper after which you cook for a minute. Transfer to a big bowl and add the other stuff. Toss gently to mix thoroughly.

**Did you know?**

*Avocados are among the healthiest foods because they contain 25+ essential nutrients and up to 15 health benefits.*

## 37. Linguine with Fresh Tomato Sauce

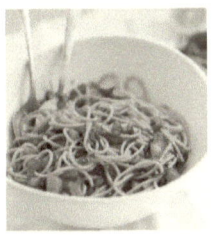

**Ingredients**

- 3 tablespoon virgin olive oil
- 3 minced garlic cloves
- I small onion, sliced
- 3 cups chopped tomatoes
- 1¼ teaspoon salt
- 12 ounces linguine
- ¼ cup grated parmesan

**Method**

1. Heat 2 tablespoons oil and cook onion over low heat for 8 minutes, stirring to ensure no burning. Add garlic and cook for a minute more. Add tomatoes and salt and stir slightly, allow to simmer for ten minutes. Cook pasta as per instructions on packet. Add to sauce and cook for a minute. Add remaining oil and toss. Top with cheese before serving.

**Did you know?**

*Eating cheese in moderation helps prevent tooth decay and protects enamel like most tooth pastes.*

## 38. Spaghetti Bolognaise

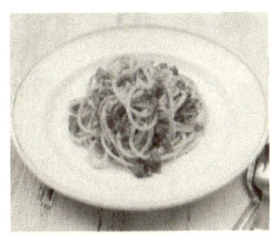

## Ingredients

- 1 tablespoon olive oil
- 200g beef mince
- 1 small onion, sliced
- A chopped garlic clove
- 50g grated carrots
- 400g tin chopped tomatoes
- 200ml beef stock
- 200g spaghetti
- Salt and pepper

## Method

1. Heat a little oil and fry mince over low heat until browned. Remove from pan and add remaining oil, fry onions until softened. Add garlic and seasoning then fry for two more minutes.

2. Add carrot, mince and tomatoes, stir well to mix. Stir in stock and allow to simmer gently. Cook pasta according to packet instructions. When pasta is cooked, drain and add to sauce and mix well.

## Did you know?

*Tomato is not a vegetable but a fruit. It contains anthocyanin which helps you keep your memory sharp and fully focused.*

## 39. Pesto Fried Pasta with Chicken

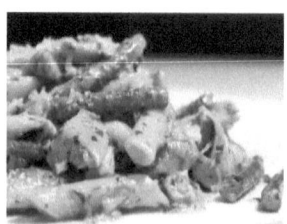

Chicken is a nutritious meat which is low in fat but high in protein and low in calories.

## Ingredients

- 5 ounces chicken breasts
- 1½ tablespoon vegetable oil

- 2 onions, chopped
- Small carrot, julienned
- Small beaten egg
- 2½ cups cold cooked macaroni elbows
- 2 tablespoons pesto sauce
- 1 teaspoon chili paste
- 1 tablespoon soy sauce

**Method**

1. Cut chicken into thin strips. Heat oil in large skillet over high heat. Put chicken, onions, carrot and chili sauce and stir-fry until chicken is cooked. Add egg and stir gently until firm. Stir in pasta and cook until heated through. Add sauces and remove from heat and mix everything well.

**Fun fact**

*Chickens can't taste sweetness in foods but can detect salt and most choose to avoid it.*

## 40. Pasta with Broccoli

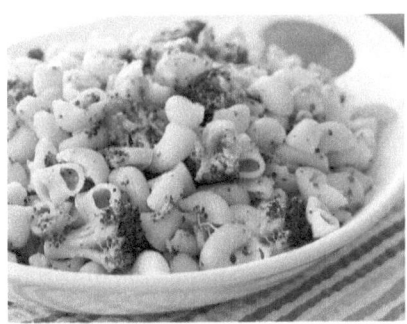

**Ingredients**

- 400g short pasta
- 5 tablespoon olive oil
- 800g broccoli florets
- 2 finely chopped garlic cloves
- 1 chili pepper, dried
- Parmesan cheese
- Salt and pepper

**Method**

1. Use method on packet to cook pasta. Meanwhile, heat oil in a thick based pan and cook florets and chili for two minutes. Add garlic and cook for a minute. Toss sauce with drained pasta, a little black pepper and cheese.

**Did you know?**

*The Chinese are believed to have eaten pasta as early as 5000 B.C.*

## 41. Italian Beef Curry & Pasta

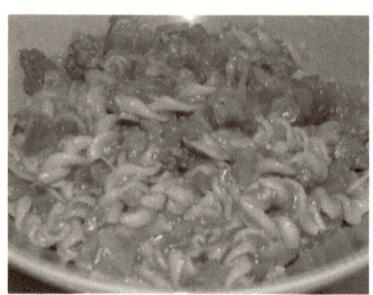

**Ingredients**

- 1-pound whole wheat macaroni
- 4 teaspoons red/green Italian curry paste
- 14 ounces can coconut milk
- 3 tablespoons fish sauce
- 2 pounds steak or chuck roast in sizable pieces
- 8 ounces mushrooms
- Medium onion and carrot both sliced thinly
- 10 ounces cauliflower florets
- 2 teaspoons salt
- ½ teaspoon pepper
- 12 ounces trimmed fresh green beans

**Method**

1. Whisk the paste, milk and sauce in the slow cooker. Add remaining ingredients except beans and stir to ensure sauce coats everything. Add beans but do not mix. Cook on low heat for 8 hours, in the last 30 minutes, stir in beans at ten-minute intervals.

2. Cook pasta according to packet instructions in the last 15 minutes before curry is done. Put drained pasta on a serving dish and top with curry.

**Did you know?**

*Mushrooms are some of the oldest living vegetables and have been used as medicine for thousands of years.*

## 42. Spaghetti with Marinara Sauce

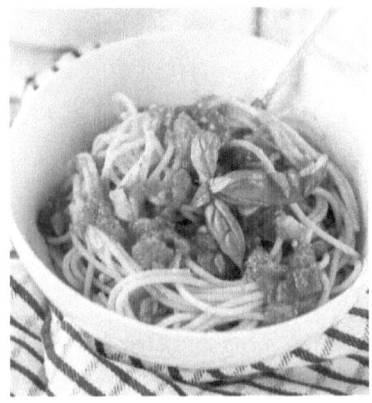

**Ingredients**

- 1-pound spaghetti
- 4 minced garlic cloves
- 2 tablespoons virgin olive oil
- 28 ounces diced tomatoes
- 1 chopped onion
- Salt and pepper

**Method**

1. Heat oil in a saucepan and fry onion over medium heat. Stir at intervals until onion becomes tender. Add garlic and cook for one more minute, stirring. Add in tomatoes and their juice and allow to boil.

2. Reduce heat and cook for a further 20 minutes then add salt and pepper. Cook spaghetti as per packet instructions and drain. Toss spaghetti with sauce and serve.

**Did you know?**

*Olive oil is rich in the anti-oxidant hydroxytyrosol. Anti-oxidants help protect the body against the damage caused by free radicals.*

### 43. Pasta Salad Ala Daniella

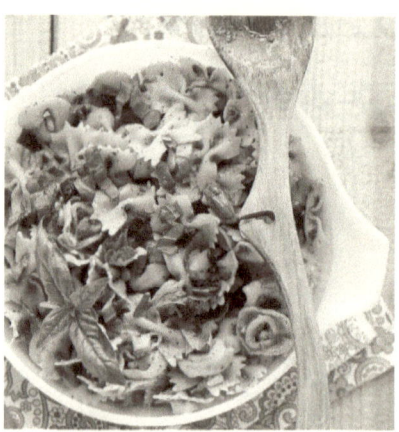

This dish is as mouth-watering, tasty and classy as the name implies.

**Ingredients**

- 1-pound pasta of choice
- 8 ounces Italian dressing
- ½ pound pepperoni, cut into small pieces
- 1 chopped cucumber
- 1 jar green olives, sliced
- 4 chopped tomatoes

**Method**

1. Cook pasta in a large pot with a lot of salted water. When tender but firm, drain and allow to cool. Place in a large bowl and add the rest of the ingredients. Toss well to mix. Cover and chill overnight if you can.

**Did you know?**

*Tomato is not a vegetable but a fruit. It contains anthocyanin which helps you keep your memory sharp and fully focused.*

## 44. Black Olives Pasta Salad

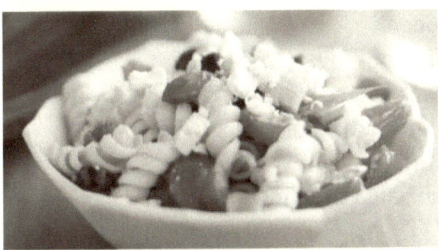

**Ingredients**

- 1 pound cooked, colored rotini pasta
- 16-ounce bottle Italian salad dressing
- ¾ jar salad seasoning, supreme
- 1 Bermuda onion, chopped
- 20 black olives, sliced and drained

**Method**

1. Mix the olives and onion well. Add the pasta and toss gently. Add seasoning and toss slightly then chill and serve.

**Did you know?**

*In the 13th century, the Roman Pope then set quality standards for pasta.*

## 45. Italian Pasta Salad

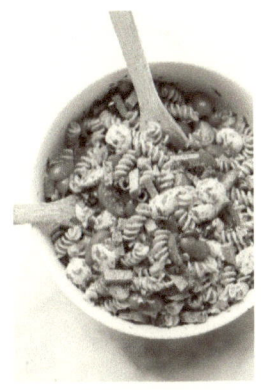

A scrumptious and filling salad the Italian way.

### Ingredients

- 1-pound broccoli
- 6 ounces tomatoes, quartered
- 20 sliced black olives
- 1 sliced and peeled cucumber
- 8 ounces rotini pasta
- ½ cup Italian salad dressing

### Method

1. Cook pasta in a lot of water until tender but firm. Drain and set aside. As pasta boils, cut broccoli and cucumber into small pieces. Drain olives. Mix all ingredients and add dressing. Chill for 30 minutes before you serve.

### Pasta Fun Fact

*Tripolini (little bows) was named to honor the Italian conquest of Tripoli.*

## 46. Confetti Spaghetti Salad

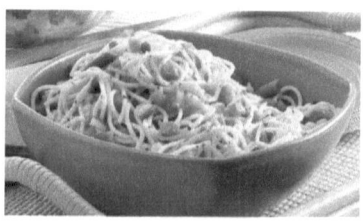

This is an appetizing dish with a colorful appeal.

### Ingredients

- 7 ounces packet spaghetti, uncooked and broken into thirds
- 2 cups frozen mixed vegetables
- ¼ cup red onion, chopped
- ¾ cup chopped tomato
- ½ cup Italian dressing

### Method

1. Boil spaghetti in a large saucepan with a lot of water and add frozen vegetables in last five minutes. Drain and allow to cool. In a medium

sized bowl, toss all ingredients gently. Cover salad and refrigerate for 45 minutes to an hour before serving.

**Did you know?**

*There are more than 600 pasta shapes produced worldwide.*

## 47. Aubergine & Ricotta Pasta

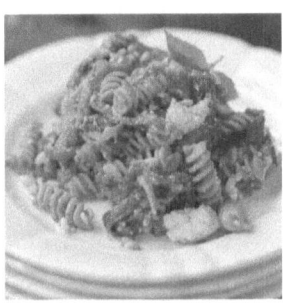

**Ingredients**

- 3 aubergines
- 10 ounces can diced tomatoes
- 12 fresh basil leaves
- Some olive oil
- 8 ounces ricotta cheese
- 2 squashed cloves of garlic
- 10 ounces pasta

**Method**

1. Slice eggplant into thin discs and use a little olive oil to grill them in the oven. Cook pasta according to instructions on packet and drain. Heat olive oil in saucepan and fry garlic, making sure not to burn it.

2. Add tomato and cook for 3 minutes. Add salt and pepper then add in torn basil leaves. Warm a bowl and use to combine and toss all the stuff. Remove garlic. Squirt raw olive oil before serving.

**Did you know?**

*Eating cheese in moderation helps prevent tooth decay and protects enamel like most tooth pastes.*

## 48. Cold Pasta Salad

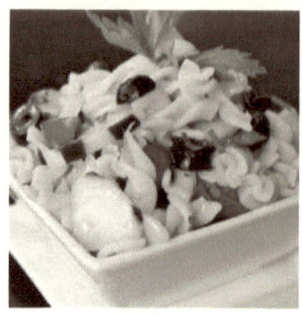

**Ingredients**

- 4 ounces uncooked pasta
- ½ cucumber, chopped
- 1/4 finely chopped onion
- 3 quartered cherry tomatoes
- 3 tablespoons pitted black olives, sliced
- 4 tablespoons Italian salad dressing

**Method**

1. Boil pasta in salted water until tender but firm. Drain and allow to cool. Combine pasta with all ingredients except salad dressing and mix well. Put the salad dressing and combine well. Cover and refrigerate for about an hour and half before you serve.

**Did you know?**

*The Chinese are believed to have eaten pasta as early as 5000 B.C.*

## 49. Almonds, Ricotta & Wilted Green Pizza

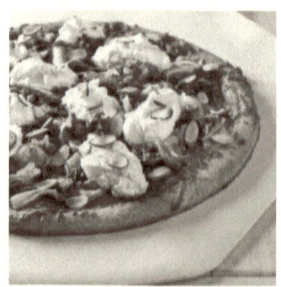

Every bit of this pizza is super healthy which is due to the fiber-filling and highly satisfying protein combo of escarole, toasted almonds and creamy ricotta.

**Ingredients**

- ¼ cup with additional 2 teaspoons of water
- 2 thinly sliced garlic cloves
- ½ teaspoon of fresh/dried rosemary(chopped)
- 1 ½ cup of escarole. Wash and slice it into ribbons with ½ inch wide
- 2 teaspoons of olive oil
- 1 cup of semi-skimmed ricotta cheese
- ¼ teaspoon of sea salt
- ¼ teaspoon of black pepper
- ¼ cup tomato paste
- 3 tablespoons of almonds (sliced)

**Method**

1. Preheat the oven to about 500 degrees. Take a large size skillet, add ¼ cup water, rosemary and garlic and boil it. Then throw in a few handfuls of escarole.

2. Cover it up and cook for about 5 minutes until they get tender. Drain the water after that. Whisk oil in a small bowl with the other 2 teaspoons of water. Brush it onto the pizza shell and then place it on a baking sheet. Put it in the oven for baking for 5 minutes and in the meantime, mix pepper, salt and ricotta in a bowl. Remove the pizza and also lower the temperature of the oven to 375 degrees.

3. Now spread the pizza crust along with the tomato paste. Top it up with ricotta and escarole mixture. Sprinkle the almond slices over it. Bake it again for a maximum of 5 minutes until the crust gets crispier and the almonds brown.

**Ricotta – The Healthiest of All the Cheeses**

*It serves as a healthy yet tasty ingredient in your pizza. It is known for its exceptional amount of proteins. It provides a good source of calcium as well.*

## 50. Maple & 3-Cheese Pear Pizza

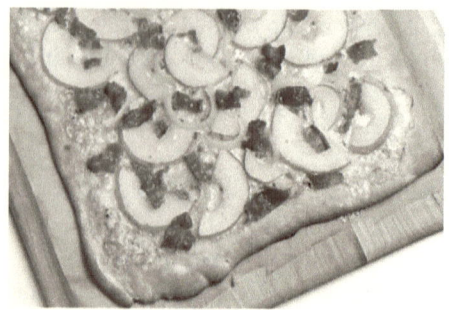

Thanks to the hemp seeds, savory cheeses and the sweet pears, this makes it one of tasty yet healthy pizzas that you can ever enjoy.

## Ingredients

- Cooking spray
- Flour (as needed)
- Pizza dough (1 pound at room temperature)
- 2 tablespoons of hemp seeds
- 1 ½ tablespoons of Parmigiano-Reggiano cheese (finely grated)
- 2 tablespoons of mozzarella cheese
- 2 tablespoons of ricotta cheese
- 3 Bosc pears (thinly sliced)
- ½ tablespoon lemon juice
- ½ tablespoon maple syrup

## Method

1. Preheat oven till 450 degrees. Line up a rimmed 16x12 inches of baking sheet along with foil and coat it using the cooking spray. Stretch fit the dough into a rectangular shape onto the baking sheet.

2. Take a bowl and mix Parmigiano-Reggiano cheese along with hemp seeds. Sprinkle it all over the dough. Then scatter the mozzarella cheese over the dough and dot it with the ricotta cheese.

3. Place the pears over the dough side by side and in 4 vertical layers; press them into the dough as well. Drizzle the partially ready dough with maple syrup and lemon juice. Then you need to bake it for 15 – 20 minutes until you notice the crust getting golden brown.

## 3-Cheese Combo Benefits

*Ricotta cheese is good with its calcium quantity. Parmigiano-Reggiano contains Vitamin A which is healthy for skin. Mozzarella cheese contains vitamin B6 benefits.*

## 51. Roasted Vegetable Pizza

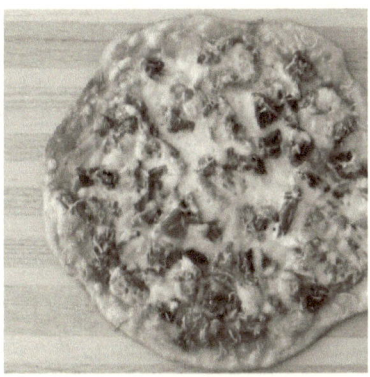

It is not only the cheese that can make an irresistible tasty pizza. This cheese-free pizza comes with red bell pepper, artichoke hearts, zucchini and black olives as the main ingredients.

## Ingredients

- 28 ounces can of drained artichoke hearts, cut in half
- 1 piece of red bell pepper, chopped into small bite-size pieces
- 1 piece of zucchini, chopped into quarter slices
- 2 pieces of minced garlic groves
- 1 tablespoon olive oil
- ¾ teaspoon of sea salt
- 1-pound pizza dough (whole wheat)
- 1 teaspoon of dried basil
- ½ cup of almond meal
- 1 teaspoon of dried oregano
- 2 pieces of tomato
- ½ cup of flour
- ½ cup of black olives (sliced)

## Method

1. Get the oven ready by preheating it to 400 degrees. Take a 9x13 inch baking pan and add ball pepper, garlic and artichoke hearts in it. Drizzle olive oil and sprinkle ¼ tsp of salt. Stir it well and then bake it for 40

minutes until you see the vegetables getting brown. Wait 20 minutes until the pizza dough gets along with the room temperature.

2. For the sauce, take a small dry skillet and toast almond meal, oregano, basil and a ¼ tsp of salt. Stir well until you achieve a thick brown sauce. Let it cool down for a few minutes. Then add the blended tomato into the mixture.

3. Roll out the dough in a 12-inch pie and preheat the oven to be at 425 degrees. Spread the prepared sauce over the dough. Top it up with roasted veggies and the olives. Bake it for 15 minutes until the flat bread gets golden brown.

**Have it with Garlic Sauce**

*The roasted vegetable pizza is best served with garlic sauce. Garlic sauce is all healthy with ingredients such as yogurt, lemon juice and garlic, etc. You can easily prepare it at home in 5 minutes.*

### 52. White Party Pizzette

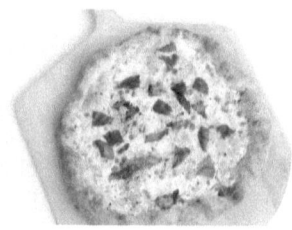

This White Party Pizzette will be a real treat for your taste buds and that too in a healthy way. It has rich vegetable ingredients such as cauliflower, chives and rosemary, which will also make it a yummy endeavor.

**Ingredients**

- 1 ½ cups of cauliflower florets, chopped into bite-size
- 1 tablespoon olive oil
- 1 ½ teaspoons of white truffle oil
- 1 minced garlic clove
- 2 teaspoons of chives (minced)
- ½ teaspoon chopped rosemary
- 1/8 teaspoon of sea salt
- 1/8 teaspoon of freshly ground white or black pepper.
- 1/8 teaspoon of dried pepper flakes

- 2 pieces of pitas or flat breads.
- ¼ cup with 2 additional teaspoons of provolone cheese (sliced)
- 1 tablespoon of grated Parmigiano-Reggiano cheese

**Method**

1. Preheat the oven to reach 450 degrees temperature. Take a bowl and mix cauliflower, truffle oil, olive oil, rosemary, chives, hot pepper flakes, black pepper and salt.

2. Top up each pita slice with equal portions of the cauliflower mixture, Parmigiano-Reggiano and the provolone cheese. Place the pitas over a baking sheet and bake until the cauliflower pieces become tender and the crust becomes crispier. Wait 5 minutes to cool down before serving.

**The Extra-Veggie Pizza Toppings**

*If you are a veggie pizza lover then there are so many toppings that will make your pizza even more irresistible. For this one, sprinkle finely chopped parsley, black olives and baked mushrooms over it for a much healthier and tasty pizza.*

### 53. Green Salad Pizza

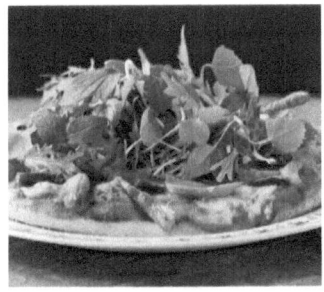

It is an open secret that green salad is rich in iron, vitamins and minerals, which puts the Green Salad Pizza on the top all the healthy pizza charts.

**Ingredients**

- 2 tablespoons of cornmeal
- 14 ounces of pizza dough (whole meat)
- 1/3 cup of marinara sauce
- 1 ½ teaspoons of dried oregano
- 1 cup plant based cheese
- 2 cups of leafy greens

- 1 ½ cups of halved cherry tomatoes
- Diced bell pepper (half)
- 1 sliced avocado
- ¼ cup of roasted pistachios
- 1 tablespoon vinegar (balsamic)
- 1 tablespoon olive oil

**Method**

1. Preheat oven at 350 degrees. Sprinkle cornmeal on a 14-inch pizza pan. Roll out the dough smoothly over the pan. Apply marinara sauce over it and sprinkle it with cheese and oregano.

2. Bake the pizza for about half an hour until you notice a golden crisp on the dough. Top the pizza with greens, bell pepper, pistachios, tomatoes and avocado after removing it from the oven. Then, drizzle it with olive oil and vinegar just when you are ready to serve.

**3 Perks of Plant based cheese**

*It is a rich source of protein. It contains vitamin B6 and biotin in good proportions. The presence of calcium makes it ideal for bones.*

### 54. Veggie Polenta Pizza

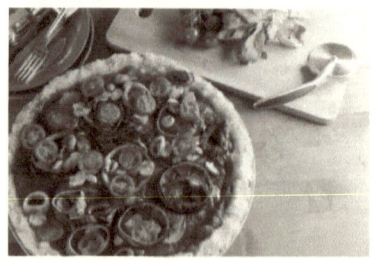

People on veggie diet will find this to be an excellent addition to their diet. This mini pizza replaces the conventional crust and comes with polenta and a range of vegetables to give you a healthier change.

**Ingredients**

- ½ cup olive oil
- 1/3 cup unsalted pistachios (roasted)
- 2 peeled garlic cloves
- ½ teaspoon of salt

- 4 cups basil (chopped)
- ½ cup Parmesan cheese (shredded)
- Cooking spray
- ½ teaspoon of black pepper
- 6 x ¼ inch thick slices of polenta
- ½ piece tomato (6 thin slices)
- ¾ cup mix vegetable (broccoli, asparagus and green beans)
- ½ cup mushrooms (sliced)
- ¾ cup of mozzarella cheese

**Method**

1. Mix garlic, olive oil, pistachios and basil in a blender until it forms a thick sauce. Add parmesan cheese and blend again. After that add pepper and salt into it. Preheat oven. Use cooking spray over a skillet set it over an average –high heat. Put the 6 polenta slices in the skillet and cook them for 3 minutes until they get golden brown.

2. After removing the golden-brown polentas, spray the skillet again with some cooking spray. Add mushrooms into it and cook for 3 minutes and make sure you stir it constantly. Top up each polenta slice with 1 tomato slice, dash pepper, pesto, mozzarella and some vegetable mix. Cook them again until the cheese melts, which will take about 5 minutes.

**Digestive Benefits of Parmesan cheese**

*It puts less strain on the metabolism. Proteins break down into its constituents very easily. Excellent amount of amino acids.*

## 55. Hula Pizza

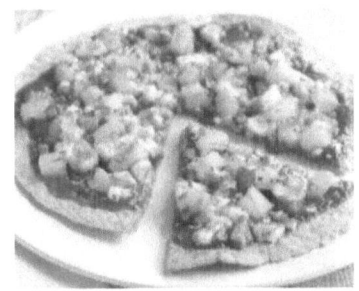

This pizza is a treat for the thin crust lovers. It has all the healthy ingredients that are enriched with proteins such as the goat cheese, pineapple and the low-fat tortilla (whole wheat).

**Ingredients**

- 1 low-fat tortilla (whole wheat)
- 2 tablespoons of barbecue sauce
- 3 tablespoons of goat cheese (crumbled)
- 3 tablespoons of diced canned pineapple (in juice)
- 1 ½ teaspoons of cilantro (chopped)

**Method**

1. Preheat oven and set the temperature at 400 degrees. Take a nonstick baking sheet and place the tortilla over it. Bake it on both sides for a couple of minutes until it becomes crispier.

2. Remove it from the oven and evenly top it with sauce, cilantro, pineapple and goat cheese. Bake it again for a maximum of 4 minutes until the goat cheese is totally melted down.

**General Tips for Healthier Pizza**

*Only add the good stuff after baking/toasting the crust. Preheating till the appropriate temperature is essential so as to avoid a soggy middle, which can cause it to be a little harder to digest. For thin crust pizzas, never overload with the toppings.*

## 56. Flatbread Pizza

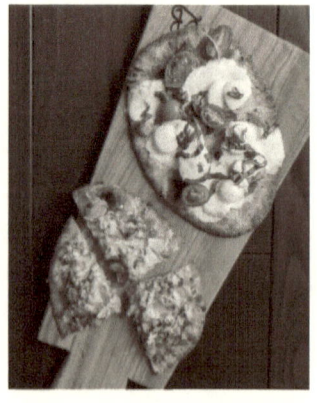

This pizza is high in fiber with the variety of veggies used, such as spinach, mushrooms and even broccoli. You have the liberty to add lean meat as well, which will give you a good amount of protein.

**Ingredients**

- 1-piece tortilla or flatbread (whole grain)
- ¼ cup of marinara sauce
- A handful of spinach leaves
- 4 sliced mushrooms
- 2 chopped broccolis
- ¼ cup of low fat mozzarella
- Oregano (Dried)
- Red pepper flakes (Dried)

**Method**

1. Preheat the oven and set it at 350 degrees. Lay the baking tray with the flatbread and spread sauce evenly. Top it up with all the vegetables in the ingredients and sprinkle it with mozzarella cheese.

2. Add red pepper and oregano according to taste. Place it in the over and toast for a maximum of 4 minutes until the cheese gets bubbly and melted.

**Top 3 Sauces that Goes Well with This Healthy Pizza**

*Garlic Coconut Cream, Hummus, and Refried bean sauce.*

## 57. Sassy Mediterranean Pizza

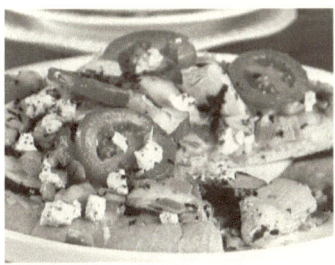

This is a healthy pizza, suitable for gluten-allergic individuals as well. It is a rare combination, but here it comes with some exceptionally healthy veggies, herbs and garlic.

## Ingredients

- 2 tablespoons of cornmeal
- 2 tablespoons of bean flour
- 1 tablespoon of flaxseed (grounded)
- ½ tablespoon of Italian herb mix (salt-free)
- 1/8 teaspoon of salt
- Cooking spray
- ½ cup of rinsed and drained cannellini beans
- 1 tablespoon olive oil
- 2 tablespoons of red onion (minced)
- ½ teaspoon of garlic (minced)
- 4 chopped basil leaves
- ¼ cup of sliced grape tomatoes
- 1 handful of mixed greens (organic)
- ½ tablespoon vinegar (balsamic)

## Method

1. Preheat the oven at 350 degrees. Mix together bean flour, flaxseed, cornmeal, salt, herb mix and 2 tablespoons of water to form a dough. Take an aluminum foil and spray it with cooking spray. Spread the dough and pat it nicely to form around crust. Bake it for 6 minutes until it gets golden and then remove it from the oven.

2. Now mash beans and mix it with garlic, onion, basil and olive oil. Spread the crust base with tomatoes and beans. Bake it again for 10 minutes and then top it with greens and drizzle some balsamic vinegar before serving.

## Top 3 Benefits of Gluten Free Pizza

*It saves you from celiac disease. It saves you from getting malnourished. It is easier to digest.*

## 58. Bean-Veggie Pizza

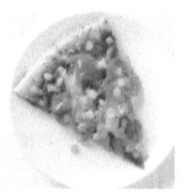

**Ingredients**

- 2 tablespoons of cornmeal
- 2 tablespoons of bean flour
- 1 tablespoon of flaxseed (grounded)
- ½ tablespoon of Italian herb mix (salt-free)
- 1/8 teaspoon of salt
- Cooking spray
- ½ cup of rinsed and drained cannellini beans
- 1 tablespoon olive oil
- 2 tablespoons of red onion (minced)
- ½ teaspoon of garlic (minced)
- 4 chopped basil leaves
- ¼ cup of sliced grape tomatoes
- 1 handful of mixed greens (organic)
- ½ tablespoon vinegar (balsamic)

**Method**

1. Preheat the oven at 350 degrees. Mix together bean flour, flaxseed, cornmeal, salt, herb mix and 2 tablespoons of water to form a dough. Take an aluminum foil and spray it with cooking spray. Spread the dough and pat it nicely to form around crust. Bake it for 6 minutes until it gets golden and then remove it from the oven.

2. Now mash beans and mix it with garlic, onion, basil and olive oil. Spread the crust base with tomatoes and beans. Bake it again for 10 minutes and then top it with greens and drizzle some balsamic vinegar before serving.

**Top 3 Benefits of Gluten Free Pizza**

*It saves you from celiac disease. It saves you from getting malnourished. It is easier to digest.*

## 59. Tomato Cheesy Pizza

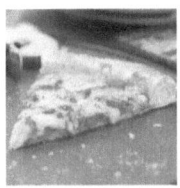

**Ingredients**

- 1 quinoa polenta tube
- 1 tablespoon of olive oil
- 3 sliced Roma tomatoes
- ½ cup mozzarella
- 3 tablespoons of chopped basil

**Method**

1. Pour some oil in the pan and heat. Cut polenta into 15 quarter inch pieces in thickness. Place it in the pan and cook properly from both sides. Preheat the oven at 350 degrees. Place polenta on an aluminum foil. Top up each piece with tomato, basil and cheese. Bake for 15minutes and it is ready.

**Top 3 Unbelievable Benefits of Tomato**

*It helps in maintaining the blood sugar level. It neutralizes and hence eliminate fats from the body. The presence of vitamin C in tomatoes reduces stress levels.*

### 60. Sweet Potato Pizza

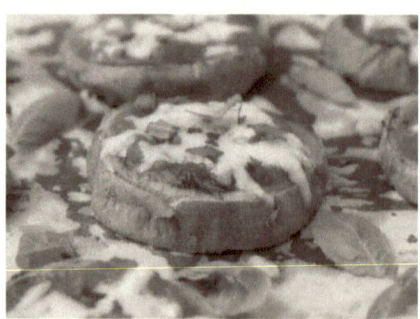

**Ingredients**

- 2 potatoes (sweet)
- 1 cup of almond flour
- 1 teaspoon of baking soda
- 1 tablespoon of seasoning (Italian)
- 1 teaspoon of salt
- ½ cup of mozzarella cheese

**Method**

1. Prepare your oven at 400 degrees and set a pot of water to boil. Add potatoes to the boiling water and boil them for 20 minutes. Drain and then mash the potatoes.

2. Take a bowl and add 1 cup of sweet mashed potato, baking soda, almond flour, salt and Italian seasoning. Apply and press the dough on a baking pan with an aluminum foil. Bake it for 20 minutes. After removing it from the oven, top it up with cheese, sauce and healthy toppings of your choice. Bake again until the cheese melts.

**Reasons That Potato is a Healthy Diet**

*It is a fat free natural food. It has a high index rating for glycemic. It is an excellent source of fiber.*

### 61. Low Carb Crust Pizza

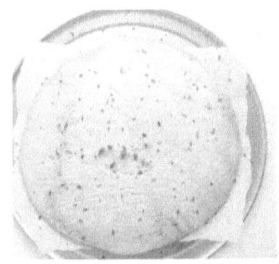

This pizza comes with a cauliflower crust and it is extremely low in carbohydrates and calories.

**Ingredients**

- Cooking spray
- 2 ½ cups of cauliflower
- 1 beaten egg
- 1 1/4 cups of mozzarella cheese
- 2 tablespoons of parmesan cheese
- Salt
- Black pepper
- ¼ cup of tomato sauce
- 2 sliced garlic cloves
- ¼ teaspoon of crushed red pepper

## Method

1. Preheat oven at 425 degrees and prepare a baking pan with a parchment paper. Grate the cauliflower until you get 2 cups of crumbles. Microwave it for 5 minutes so that it becomes soft.

2. Take a bowl and mix egg, parmesan cheese, mozzarella, salt and pepper. Once the mixture is ready, then pat it in the prepared pizza tray. Bake for 15 minutes. After removing the pizza, top it with sauce and some extra mozzarella. Garlic, red flakes and grape tomato should also be added. Bake again until the cheese melts.

### Nutritional Facts About the Low Carb Crust Pizza

*It will give you 272 calories per serving of 400 grams. Total fats per serving will be just 14.5 grams. The amount of cholesterol will be only 128mg.*

## 62. Chickpea Crust Pizza

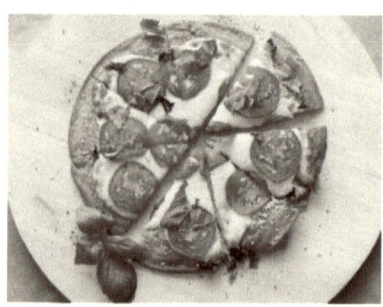

The chickpea crust pizza is gluten free with enough protein as some meaty pizzas. It is ideal for people who have a gluten allergy and holds several other health benefits as well with its rich ingredients.

### Ingredients

- 2 tablespoons cornmeal
- 2 tablespoons bean flour
- Cooking spray
- 1 tablespoon flaxseed (grounded)
- ½ tablespoon of Italian herb mix
- 1/8 teaspoon of salt

**Method**

1. Mix all the ingredients in a bowl to form a dough. Take an aluminum foil and put it over the pizza pan with cooking spray on it. Spread and press well the pizza dough in an even manner.

2. In a preheated oven at 350 degrees, bake it for about 6 minutes until you see the crust getting golden. Remove it from the oven and serve it with your favorite toppings.

**Top 3 Healthiest Toppings for This Pizza**

*Goat Cheese Crumbles, Arugula, and Rosemary Marinara Sauce.*

## 63. Veggie Gluten-Free Mini Pizza

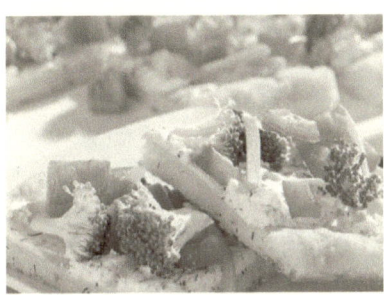

These small size pizzas are excellent for their extremely low calories and carbohydrates. It is gluten-free as well, which makes it ideal for the health conscious and gluten-allergic individuals.

**Ingredients**

- 4 small slices of gluten free pizza crusts
- 13 ounces of tomato sauce
- 1 cup mozzarella cheese
- 1 cup chopped tomatoes
- 1 cup of chopped green and red peppers
- ½ cup of mushrooms
- 1 cup of spinach leaves
- ½ cup finely chopped onions
- 3 tablespoons of olive oil
- 1 teaspoon of salt
- 2 teaspoons of black pepper

**Method**

1. Preheat the oven at 375 degrees. Take a bowl and add chopped tomatoes with salt, black pepper and olive oil and mix it well. Take a cookie sheet and place the pizza crust over it. Bake it for 5 minutes each for both sides.

2. Apply tomato sauce on each crust. Then sprinkle cheese and all other vegetables in equal amount and evenly. Bake it again for 20 minutes.

**The Top 3 Spinach Health Benefits**

*The presence of lutein in spinach is good for the eyes. It fights cholesterol. Spinach has lots of iron and fiber.*

## 64. Quinoa Pizza Bites

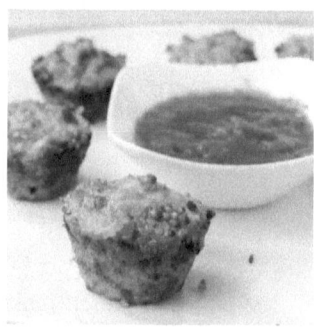

Quinoa is an excellent ingredient for a pizza to make it highly nutritious treat. It's also packed with lots of fiber and protein.

**Ingredients**

- 1 cup of quinoa (uncooked)
- 2 eggs
- 1 cup mozzarella cheese
- 2 teaspoons of garlic paste
- ½ cup of chopped basil
- ½ cup of diced tomatoes
- ½ teaspoon of salt
- 1 teaspoon of paprika
- 1 teaspoon of oregano

**Method**

1. Boil quinoa in a covered pot and simmer it until it becomes tender. Preheat the oven at 350 degrees. Mix all the given ingredients in a bowl.

2. Take a cookie sheet and add all the mixture properly into the shaped pots. Bake it for a maximum of 20 minutes and serve it after cooling it down for 10 minutes.

**The Exceptional Health Perks of Quinoa**

*Quinoa is known to be naturally gluten free. It is a good source of iron, Vitamin B & E, magnesium, fiber and calcium. It contains nine essential amino acids.*

### 65. Strawberry Arugula Pizza

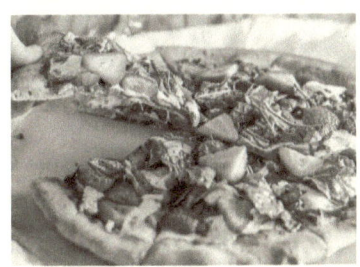

**Ingredients**

- ½ sliced basil
- ¾ cup of sliced strawberries
- 1 tablespoon of olive oil
- 3 ounces goat cheese
- 2 teaspoons of vinegar
- ½ cup of sliced arugula
- 2 ounces pizza dough
- Black pepper (as needed)

**Method**

1. Preheat the oven at about 450 degrees. Roll and spread the dough over the pizza pan. Using a pastry brush, brush over the crust with olive oil and a single teaspoon of vinegar. Bake it in the oven for 5 minutes.

2. Remove it and top it with basil, strawberries, arugula and cheese. Bake it again for 10 minutes and let the crust get light brown in color.

## How Strawberries Help Your Body

*Strawberries keeps a good check on your blood glucose level. They are stuffed with highly productive disease fighting antioxidants. The nutritional profile of strawberries is excellent with a reasonable amount of calories and good amount of fiber as well.*

### 66. Mini Mexican Pizza

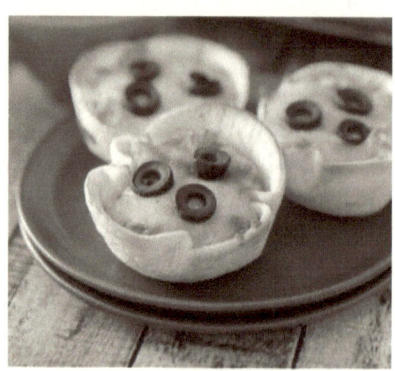

**Ingredients**

- 4 tortillas, cut into 12 smaller pieces
- 1 cup of turkey (lean ground)
- ½ cup of salsa
- 2 teaspoons of taco seasoning
- ½ cup of refried beans
- ½ cup of cheddar cheese

**Method**

1. Preheat the oven at about 425 degrees. Spray a 12-pocket cookie sheet with cooking spray. Place each of the small tortilla pieces in the cookie tray using your finger.

2. Take a bowl and mix taco seasoning, refried beans, salsa and ground turkey meat into it. Scoop an equal amount of mixture into each pot and top it up with cheese. Bake it in the oven for 15 minutes or when you notice the cheese melting.

**Top 3 Optional Toppings for the Mini Mexican Pizza**

*Low fat sour cream spread over the pizza after it is baked. Toppings using black olives and chopped tomatoes make a great combination. The shredded lettuce topping is excellent for veggie lovers.*

## 67. Spicy Turkey Sausage Pizza

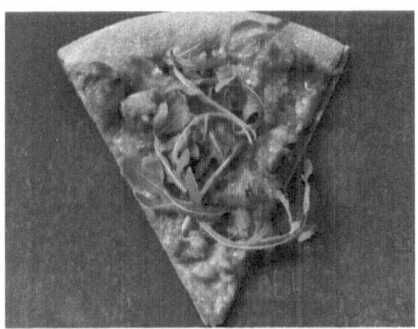

Turkey meat is high in protein and known as one of the best types of meat due to its low-fat content – so this pizza is definitely a tasty but also healthy option for the whole family.

**Ingredients**

- 1 piece of turkey sausage about 4 ounces
- Pizza crust (prebaked)
- ¾ cup of marinara sauce
- ½ cup of mozzarella cheese (semi-skimmed)
- 1 cup arugula

**Method**

1. Break the sausage into smaller pieces. Prepare a pizza pan and place the prebaked pizza crust over it. Spread it over the marinara sauce. Sprinkle the crust with the sausage and mozzarella cheese. Bake it in a preheated oven for about 10 minutes and take it out once the cheese is melted. After taking it out, top it up with arugula.

**The Unknown Benefits About Turkey Meat**

*It is a very rich source of protein. Turkey is reasonable and comparatively low in fat. Regular intake of turkey can control cholesterol levels.*

## 68. Eggplant Parmesan Pizza

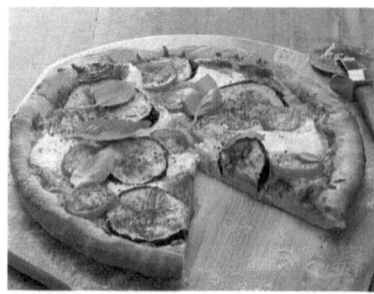

A single serving of Eggplant Parmesan Pizza contains just 8 grams of fat. It uses all-natural ingredients, which makes it one of the finest veggie pizzas for you to enjoy.

## Ingredients

- ¾ cup of marinara sauce
- Pizza dough (refrigerated)
- 2 ½ ounce of mozzarella cheese (semi-skimmed)
- ½ cup of ricotta cheese (semi-skimmed)
- 3 sliced plum tomatoes
- ¾ pound of sliced and broiled eggplant
- 1 tablespoon of Parmesan cheese
- Handful of basil leaves

## Method

1. Spread the prepared dough over the pizza pan and apply marinara sauce over it. Sprinkle the shredded mozzarella and ricotta cheese over it. Top it with plum tomatoes and the sliced eggplant.

2. Sprinkle the Parmesan cheese over it. Bake it in a preheated oven at 450 degrees for about 10 minutes until it becomes light brown. Remove it from the oven and sprinkle basil leaves before serving.

## Healthy Reasons to Eat More Eggplants

*Eggplants contain an excellent amount of photo nutrients that helps in improving blood circulation. It is rich in calcium, minerals and iron. The amount of fiber in eggplants helps people with the protection of their digestive tract.*

## 69. Black Bean Nacho Pizza

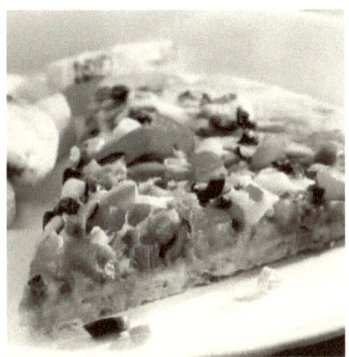

### Ingredients

- 2 ¼ teaspoons of dry yeast
- 1 teaspoon sugar
- 1 cup flour
- ½ teaspoon salt
- 2 tablespoons of cornmeal
- 1 piece of quartered garlic clove
- 1 cup Jack cheese (shredded)
- ½ cup roasted red peppers
- ¼ cup chopped black olives
- 4 pieces of medium size scallions

### Method

1. Add 2 tablespoons of lukewarm water, salt, sugar and yeast in a large bowl. After 5 minutes of waiting, add and mix thoroughly bread flour, whole-wheat flour and cornmeal to form a dough.

2. Spread the prepare dough over a pizza pan and put it in a preheated oven at 450 degrees for 3 minutes until it gets a bit crispier. Quickly add the toppings evenly over the surface of the crust. Bake it for another 15 minutes until the crust gets light brown in color.

### Nutritional Profile of Black Bean Nacho Pizza

*A single serving contains just 8g of fats. The total calories per serving is 317 calories. It contains 249mg potassium, 692mg sodium, 17mg cholesterol, 46g carbs, 17mg cholesterol and 6g fiber per serving.*

## 70. Broccoli Rabe & Chicken Pizza

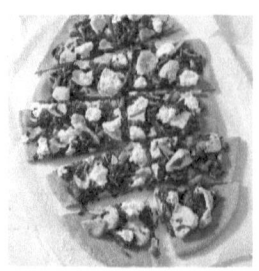

Broccoli and chicken make a very rich, healthy and tasty combination. The benefits of white meat are quite obvious with proteins and then the low-fat recipe will make it a truly healthy feast for all pizza lovers.

## Ingredients

- 1-pound prepared pizza dough
- 12 ounces of skinless and boneless chicken meat, chopped into small pieces
- 4 tablespoons of olive oil
- ¼ cup of garlic (sliced)
- 6 cups of broccoli (chopped)
- 1 tablespoon of lemon juice
- ½ teaspoon black pepper
- ¼ teaspoon of salt
- Lemon zest
- ½ cup ricotta cheese

## Method

1. Preheat the oven at a temperature of 425 degrees. Line up a baking sheet and place over the rolled dough evenly around the surface of the baking pan. Bake for about 10 minutes to make the crust crispier.

2. Put 3 tablespoons of olive oil in a skillet and heat gently. Add garlic and cook/stir for 1 minute. Add in broccoli rabe, chicken pepper, salt, lemon zest and cook well until the chicken is properly cooked.

3. Now transfer all the chicken mixture over the half-ready crust evenly. Mix lemon juice and ricotta cheese and spread it over the crust. This time bake it for about 6 – 8 minutes until the crust shows light brown color.

## Why Broccoli is So Popular Among Health-Conscious People

*The soluble fiber in broccoli helps reducing cholesterol. It acts as a very powerful antioxidant. It helps in the prevention of cancer.*

## 71. Tomato Butter Dip

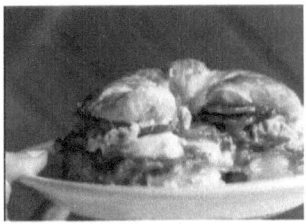

This is a great dip for veggies, chips, or chicken wings.

**Ingredients**

- Cherry Tomatoes
- Butter (softened)
- Salt

**Method**

1. Broil tomatoes until skins blister. Let it cool. Pulse together with salt in a food processor. Stir mixture into butter until well blended.

**Tomato Trivia**

*The tomato is a tricky plant. Scientifically, it is a fruit. The tomato is the state vegetable of New Jersey and the state fruit of Ohio. But Arkansas beats both: the tomato is their state fruit and state vegetable.*

## 72. Stuffed Tomatoes

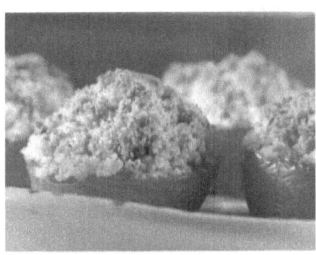

**Ingredients**

- 1 loaf Italian Bread (crust removed)
- 2 cloves Garlic (chopped)
- 2 tbsp. capers
- 2 tsp salt
- 6 tbsp. olive oil
- 4 large tomatoes

**Method**

1. Preheat oven to 250°F. Bake bread for 5 minutes on each side. Set aside. Raise temperature to 350°F. Cut bread into chunks and place in food processor. Pulse until crumbly but not pulverized. Set aside 1 cup of crumbs. Store the rest for later.

2. In a bowl, mix garlic, capers, breadcrumbs, salt, and olive oil. Halve the tomatoes and remove seeds. Fill the halves with breadcrumb mixture. Place on baking sheet. Bake for 20 minutes or until brown crust forms.

**Tomato Trivia**

*Tomatoes are native to the Andes Mountains in Peru. The Aztec of Mexico believed that the seeds gave people the ability to see the future. When it was first brought to Italy, it was thought to be poisonous. The Spanish, on the other hand, thought it was an eggplant.*

## 73. Tomato Gravy

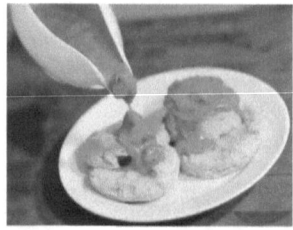

This healthier twist on gravy doesn't sacrifice flavor.

**Ingredients**

- ½ cup butter
- 2 medium onions (chopped)
- 2 tsp thyme

- 2 tbsp. flour
- 1 (28 oz.) can crushed tomatoes
- 1/3 cup scallions (sliced)
- 3 tbsp. heavy cream
- 1 tsp cayenne pepper
- Salt & pepper to taste

**Method**

1. Melt butter in a large pan on medium heat. Add thyme and onion. Cook 10 minutes, stirring often. Add flour. Cook 3 minutes, stirring constantly. Add tomatoes with juice. Cook 30 minutes. Stir in cream, cayenne, scallions, salt, and pepper.

**Tomato Trivia**

*Despite being native to South America, China has now become the largest producer of tomatoes today. Tomatoes aren't just red. They can also be orange, yellow, green, pink, purple, brown, white, or black. Today, there are more than 7,500 species of tomato.*

## 74. Tomato & Corn Salad

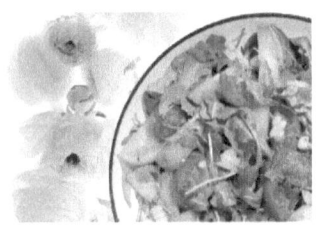

This simple salad proves that delicious doesn't have to be difficult.

**Ingredients**

- 6 large Tomatoes (diced)
- 20 ears of corn
- Salt, Pepper, Oil, Paprika to taste

**Method**

1. Prepare a grill on high heat. Blanch corn until bright yellow. Let air dry. Grill corn until slightly scorched on all sides. Remove kernels from the

cobs. Add the kernels, tomatoes, salt, pepper, and paprika to a large bowl. Stir. Add olive oil and mix until evenly coated.

**Tomato Trivia**

*In Spain, there is an annual tomato fight. Over 40,000 people gather to pelt each other with tomatoes. The Guinness World Record for the biggest tomato weighed in at a whopping 7 lbs. and 12 oz. (the size of a healthy newborn baby). A single tomato plant at the Epcot Science project in Disney World produced over 32,000 tomatoes in a single year.*

### 75. Tomato Bites

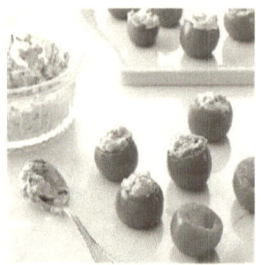

These simple yet flavorful snacks are the perfect treat for a summer day.

**Ingredients**

- 2 lbs. Tomatoes (sliced)
- 1 Scallion (sliced)
- 3 Tbsps. Olive Oil
- 2 Tbsps. Malt Vinegar
- ¾ tsp Brown Sugar
- Salt & Pepper to taste

**Method**

1. Whisk together salt, pepper, brown sugar, vinegar, and oil in a bowl. Arrange 1/3 of the tomatoes on a platter. Drizzle a little of the oil mixture over them. Sprinkle some scallions on top. Repeat process twice to make 2 more layers.

**Tomato Trivia**

*Eating a serving of tomatoes every day can reduce men's risk of prostate cancer by up to 43%. Lycopene (the nutrient responsible for the cancer fighting effects) is best absorbed in fat so make sure you drizzle on a little extra olive oil! Early research results suggest that tomatoes may even help combat the spread of cancer in patients who are already ill.*

### 76. Tomato Focaccia

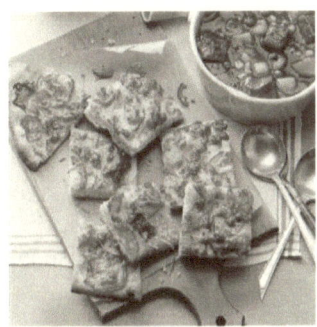

This wonderful focaccia is just the right blend of satisfyingly hearty and refreshingly light.

**Ingredients**

- ½ lbs. Potatoes (peeled, quartered)
- ½ lbs. Tomatoes (sliced)
- ½ cup Olive Oil
- 4 ¼ cups Flour
- 1 cup Warm Water
- 3 tsp Active Dry Yeast
- 1 Tbsp. Salt
- ½ tsp Sugar
- ¼ tsp Oregano

**Method**

1. Simmer potatoes in salt water for 10 to 15 minutes. Drain, cool, and mash. In a large bowl, mix sugar and warm water. Sprinkle in yeast. Let it rest 5 minutes. Add mashed potatoes and ¼ cup oil. Mix until combined.

2. Add flour 1 cup at a time and mix until a soft, sticky dough forms. Knead on a floured surface 8-10 minutes. Place an oiled bowl and cover with oiled plastic wrap. Let rest in a warm place until doubled in size.

3. Punch dough down and transfer to a greased baking dish. Stretch dough so that it covers the bottom (may not fit exactly). Preheat oven to 425°F. Arrange tomatoes on top. Sprinkle with oregano, salt and ¼ cup oil. Bake until firm and pale golden (20 to 25 minutes).

**Tomato Trivia**

*For women, the lycopene in tomato can help prevent cancer in the cervix, breasts and uterus. If you're a smoker, eat a couple extra servings of tomato per day. Lycopene also helps guard against lung cancer. Lycopene and vitamin A (both found in tomatoes) help make the skin more resistant to sun damage so make sure to eat extra in the summer.*

## 77. Watermelon Tomato Salad

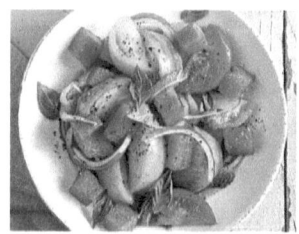

Leave your guests stunned with this mouthwateringly unique salad.

**Ingredients**

- 4 medium Tomatoes
- 1 small Cucumber
- 1 cup Watermelon (cubed)
- 1 Hass Avocado (diced)
- 3 Tbsps. Olive Oil
- 3 Tbsps. Balsamic Vinegar
- ¼ tsp Ground Coriander Seeds
- 1 Tbsp. Mixed Herbs (your preference)
- Salt & Pepper to Taste

**Method**

1. In a large bowl, combine watermelon, tomato, avocado, cucumber, herbs, and coriander. Mix well. In a small bowl, whisk together vinegar, salt, pepper, and oil. Pour vinegar mixture over tomato mixture. Toss to coat.

**Tomato Trivia**

*Americans eat an average of 24 lbs. of tomatoes each year. Over half of that amount is in the form of ketchup. That amount has increased by 30% over the past 20 years.*

## 78. Tomato Egg Cups

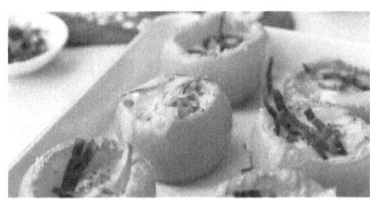

This ingenious dish makes a perfect breakfast.

**Ingredients**

- 4 medium Tomatoes
- 4 large Eggs
- 4 Tbsps. Cheddar Cheese (shredded)
- 4 slices Toast (cut in strips)
- Salt & Pepper to taste

**Method**

1. Preheat oven to 425°F. Slice the top 1/3 of each tomato. Set aside. Remove seeds. Place tomatoes in baking dish. Season with salt and pepper.

2. Crack an egg into each tomato. Put tomato tops back in place. Bake 10 minutes. Remove tops, sprinkle in cheese. Bake until bubbly (5-7 minutes). Serve with toast strips for dipping.

**Tomato Trivia**

*In German, the word for tomato (Paridiesapfel) translates to "apple of paradise." The scientific name (solanum lycopersicum) translates as "wolf peach." The word "tomato" comes from the original Aztec word xitomatl which literally translates as "plump thing with a navel."*

## 79. Tomato Gelato

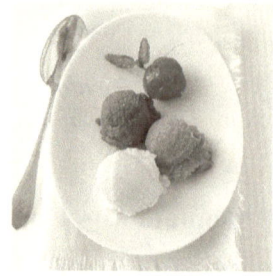

Pair this exquisite gelato with candied tomatoes and watch everyone come asking for the recipe.

**Ingredients**

- 2 lbs. Tomatoes (very ripe, chopped)
- 1 cup Simple Syrup (chilled)
- 1 pinch Salt

**Method**

1. Puree tomatoes until smooth. Strain through a fine sieve until you have 2 cups of puree. Add simple syrup and a pinch of salt. Blend well. Transfer mixture to an ice cream maker. Process according to instructions.

**Tomato Trivia**

*The acidity in tomatoes make them a perfect deep pore cleanser. Mash one up with some olive oil and give yourself a 20-minute facial. Mix a tablespoon of tomato juice with 2 drops of lime juice for a quick 10-minute pore-refining mask. Using either of these masks on a weekly basis will also help manage oily skin.*

## 80. Tomato Sliders

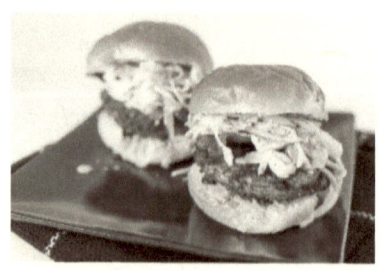

This recipe provides you with 3 different tomato-based appetizers so you're sure to please every palate.

**Ingredients**

- 8 large Tomatoes (in ½" slices)
- ¾ cup Hummus
- ¾ cup Black Olive Spread
- ¾ cup Pesto
- 2 cups Ricotta
- 3-4 Tbsps. Olive Oil
- Crusty bread
- Pepper to taste

**Method**

1. Spread hummus over 8 slices. Spread black olive spread over 8 slices. Spread pesto over 8 slices. Arrange slices on a platter. Serve with bread slices and a bowl of ricotta with pepper and olive oil drizzled on top.

**Tomato Trivia**

*A blend of tomato, aloe vera, and yogurt are the perfect homemade remedy for sunburns. Tomato juice also happens to make an excellent shampoo and conditioner. Massage it into your scalp for 5 minutes to break apart buildup and rehydrate your scalp and hair. Use a mask of tomato and honey on your face for 15 minutes to restore that natural youthful glow.*

## 81. Tomato Pudding

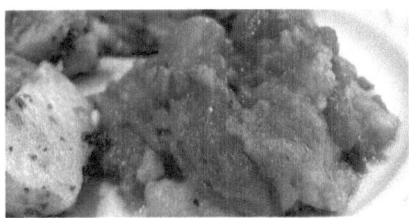

Put a new twist on tired old pudding with this savory tomato recipe.

**Ingredients**

- 4 ½ lbs. Tomatoes
- 1 (1 ¼ lbs.) Pullman Loaf (crust removed)

- 3 cloves Garlic (minced)
- 2 Tbsps. Olive Oil
- 2 ½ tsp Sherry Vinegar

**Method**

1. Blanch tomatoes for 1 minute. Remove skin. Blend garlic and salt to a paste. Halve tomatoes and remove seeds. Press seeds through a fine sieve to collect the juices. Discard seeds. Chop tomatoes and puree with collected tomato juice. Heat 2 tablespoons olive oil in a large pan on medium-high heat. Add garlic past. Cook 1 minute. Remove from heat. Add a few spoonful's puree. When no longer bubbling, add remaining puree, salt, and pepper. Return to heat. Simmer 5 minutes, stirring occasionally.

2. Cool for 1 hour. Add vinegar. Cut bread into 12 triangle pieces and 3 circular pieces. Ladle ¾ cup tomato puree into soufflé dish. Place circular bread piece at the bottom. Fan 4 triangle pieces around until puree is covered completely. Repeat layers until filled (about 3 more times). Cover top layer of bread with remaining puree. Cover with plastic wrap then place a plate just small enough to fit inside the dish on top. Weight down the pudding with 2 heavy cans or a 2 lbs. object. Chill 12 hours.

**Tomato Trivia**

*Tomatoes continue to gain weight even after being harvested. Save a few cents at the store by getting unripe tomatoes and letting them ripen (and grow) at home! In Victorian England, it was not socially acceptable to eat a tomato in public. Tomato seedlings have been successfully grown in space.*

## 82. Tomato Consommé

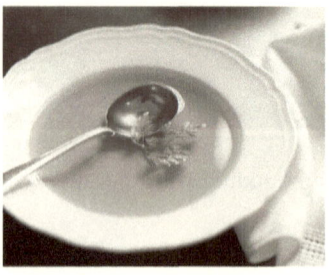

This consommé is light, refreshing, and simple to make.

**Ingredients**

- 5 lbs. Tomatoes (pureed)
- 10 oz. Pear Tomatoes (halved)
- 2 Onions (chopped)
- 1 ½ lbs. Fennel (halved lengthwise, cored, chopped)
- ¼ cup Parsley
- 8 large Egg Whites (chilled)
- 2 cloves Garlic (chopped)
- 2 Tbsps. Olive Oil
- 2 Tbsps. Basil
- 1 Tbsp. Tarragon
- ½ cup Crushed Ice
- 1 ½ tsp Sherry Vinegar

**Method**

1. In a large pot cook garlic, fennel, and onions in oil for 10-12 minutes. Stir in pureed tomato, salt, and pepper. Simmer 20 minutes. Pour mixture through a fine sieve into a large pan. Bring to a boil.

2. In a bowl, whisk together egg whites, ice, herbs, salt, and pepper until frothy. Pour egg white mixture into boiling broth, whisking constantly. Egg mixture will rise and form a "raft". Wait for the "raft" to bubble. Enlarge the holes made by bubbles to the size of a ladle.

3. Reduce heat and simmer 15-20 minutes (without stirring). Remove from heat. Ladle out consommé without disturbing the "raft". Place consommé in a fine sieve lined with damp paper towels set in a large glass bowl. Chill 1-2 hours. Before serving, toss per tomatoes with vinegar and salt. Serve on top of consommé.

**Tomato Trivia**

*The leaves of the tomato plant are toxic. The largest tomato vine is over 65 feet long. It can be found in England. The largest tomato tree can be found in Disney World but it was first discovered in Beijing.*

## 83. Tomato Snacks

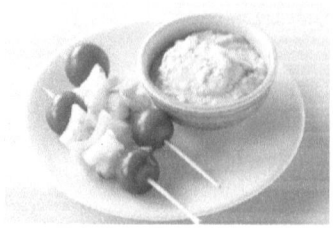

In just 10 minutes, you'll have a scrumptious snack that's ideal for summer picnics.

**Ingredients**

- 1 (8") Sourdough Round (cut into 3/4" slices)
- 4 small Tomatoes (halved)
- 2 cloves Garlic (halved)
- 4 Tbsps. Olive Oil
- Salt to taste

**Method**

1. Prepare grill for medium heat. Grill bread 1-2 minutes per side. Vigorously rub 1 side of each slice with garlic. Do the same with tomato (until most of the pulp is absorbed in the bread. Brush bread with oil and sprinkle with salt.

**Tomato Trivia**

*Storing tomatoes in the fridge makes them less nutritious and less flavorful. Keep them on the counter! The high vitamin C content in tomatoes is almost completely destroyed when cooked. However, the lycopene content is easier to digest in cooked tomatoes. So, eat a balance of raw and cooked tomatoes to get both.*

## 84. Tomato Blossoms

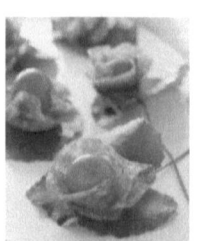

These adorable treats are easy to make and sure to put a smile on anyone's face.

**Ingredients**

- 18 Grape Tomatoes
- 18 Thin Slices Genoa Salami
- 18 long Fresh Chives
- 1/3 cup Peppered Boursin Cheese

**Method**

1. Stir basil and cheese until combined. Put ½ teaspoon of cheese mixture in the center of each salami round. Press 1 tomato into the center of each cheese pile until stabilized. Gather salami up around the tomato and tie it in place with chive.

**Tomato Trivia**

*Tomatoes are high in potassium making them a great pre-workout (or post-hangover) snack. They're also a good source of Vitamins A, K, and B vitamins (not to mention many minerals) so if you're looking for a well-rounded nutritious snack—the tomato is the answer. Lycopene also prevents wrinkles!*

## 85. Pomegranate Tomato Salad

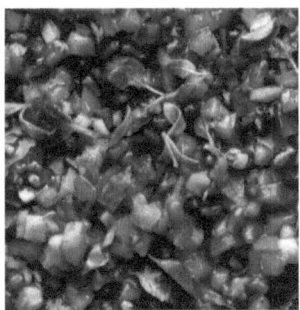

Impress your guests with this salad that's not just boldly flavored but a visually stunning masterpiece.

**Ingredients**

- 2 2/3 cups Cherry Tomatoes (red and yellow, diced)
- 1 1/3 cup Plum Tomatoes (diced)
- 1 lbs. medium Tomatoes (diced)

- 1 Red Pepper (diced)
- 1 Red Onion (diced)
- 1 cup Pomegranate Seeds
- 2 cloves Garlic (crushed)
- 1 ½ Tbsps. Molasses
- ¼ cup Olive Oil
- 2 tsp White Wine Vinegar
- 1 Tbsp. Oregano
- ½ tsp Allspice
- ½ tsp Salt

**Method**

1. In a large bowl, combine tomatoes, onion, and red pepper. In a small bowl, whisk together vinegar, molasses, garlic, olive oil, allspice, and salt. Pour this over tomato mixture and mix until evenly coated. Arrange mixture with juices on a platter. Sprinkle pomegranate seeds and oregano over the top.

**Tomato Trivia**

*The calcium and vitamin K in tomatoes help fight osteoporosis. The chromium helps stabilize blood sugar levels. The Vitamin A prevents age related macular degeneration in the eyes.*

## 86. Grilled Tomato Toasts

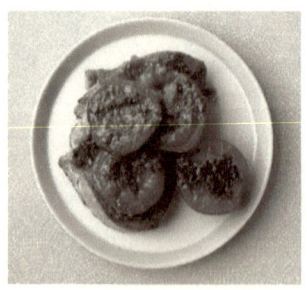

These no-hassle treats are the perfect appetizer or light lunch.

**Ingredients**

- ¾ lbs. Small Tomatoes
- 8 slices Crusty Bread
- 10 oz. Ricotta

- 1 cup Mixed Fresh Herbs (your preference)
- 1 clove Garlic (chopped)
- 6 Tbsps. Olive Oil
- 1 Tbsp. Red Wine Vinegar
- Salt & Pepper to taste

**Method**

1. Combine garlic and salt into a paste. Transfer to a bowl. Whisk in 2 tablespoons oil and the vinegar. Add tomatoes, salt, and pepper. Toss to coat. Prepare grill to medium-high heat.

2. Brush both sides of bread with olive oil. Grill 1-2 minutes per side. Add herbs to tomato mixture. Toss until evenly mixed. Spread ricotta on top of toast. Top with tomato mixture.

**Tomato Trivia**

*Getting your daily dose of tomatoes will reduce your risk for kidney stones and gallstones. Tomatoes have anti-inflammatory effects making them a great pain reliever. Tomatoes are low in calories but highly satisfying making them an excellent addition to your weight loss program.*

## 87. Oil Poached Tomatoes

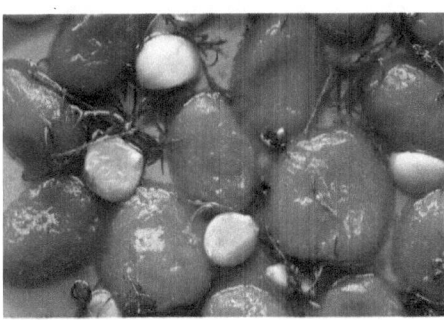

Tomatoes are the unchallenged star of this wonderfully elegant dish.

**Ingredients**

- 1 lbs. Plum Tomatoes (halved)
- 1 head Garlic (cloves separated)
- 1 cup Olive Oil
- 2 sprigs Rosemary

- 2 sprigs Thyme
- Salt to taste

**Method**

1. Preheat oven to 300°F. Toss together rosemary, garlic, oil, thyme, and salt in a baking dish. Bake tomatoes until soft (35-45 minutes). Remove skins. Discard herbs.

**Tomato Trivia**

*Tomatoes should be a big part of your diet if you're diabetic as they help your body process glucose better. The choline in tomatoes helps your body break down and absorb fat. It also helps you sleep better.*

## 88. Grilled (Tomato Prosciutto) Cheese

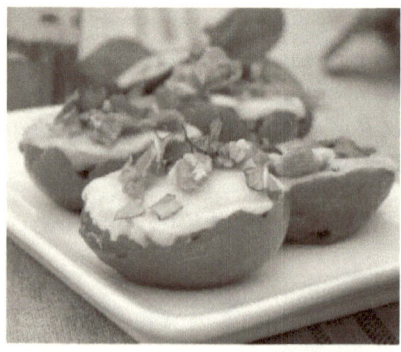

Turn that regular grilled cheese into a restaurant quality lunch with these simple modifications.

**Ingredients**

- 8 slices Whole Grain Bread
- 8 slices Prosciutto
- 2 cups Cheddar (shredded)
- ½ can Tomatoes
- 1/8 cup Red Onion (chopped)
- 4 Tbsps. Olive Oil
- 1 Tbsp. Red Wine Vinegar
- 1 clove Garlic (minced)
- ½ tsp Honey

**Method**

1. Preheat oven to 350°F. In a small pot on medium heat, cook onion, garlic, and tomato until it resembles a jam (about 15 minutes). Add honey and vinegar. Cook 15 minutes.

2. Season with salt and pepper. Remove from heat. Arrange half of your bread slices on a baking sheet. Top each slice with ¼ cup cheese and 1 slice prosciutto. Bake 3 minutes. Spread tomato jam on top of the prosciutto. Top with remaining bread slices. Heat 1 tablespoon oil in a pan. Cook each sandwich for 3 minutes per side.

**Tomato Trivia**

*The high potassium in tomatoes also helps to lower blood pressure. Fiber, potassium, and vitamin C work together to protect your heart from disease and heart attack. Tomatoes help maintain collagen in the skin and prevents damage from not only the sun but also pollution, smoke, and the aging process.*

### 89. Tomato Vinaigrette

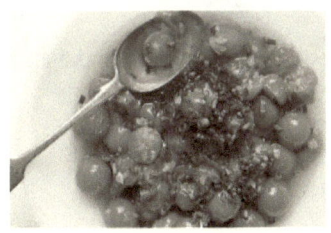

Liven up any salad with this delicious and simple vinaigrette.

**Ingredients**

- 1 lbs. Cherry Tomatoes
- 3 Tbsps. Olive Oil
- 1 Tbsp. Red Wine Vinegar
- 2 Tbsps. Chives (chopped)
- 1 Shallot (chopped)
- Salt & Pepper to taste

**Method**

1. Halve ½ lbs. cherry tomatoes. Heat 1 tablespoon oil in a pan on medium heat. Add shallot. Cook 4 minutes, stirring often. Add all the tomatoes

(halved and whole). Cook 4-6 minutes. Mash some of the tomatoes with a spoon. Add vinegar and 2 tablespoons oil. Season with salt and pepper.

**Tomato Trivia**

*Tomatoes are a great source of folic acid (especially important for pregnant women). Folic acid may also treat depression. The lycopene is even more effective than it is in other sources because, in the tomato, it's teamed up with its 3 carotenoid cousins (alpha, beta, and lutein).*

## 90. Hot Tomatoes

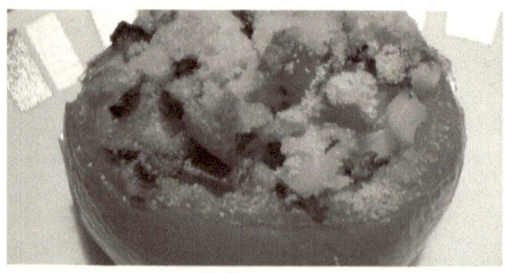

These simple yet bold appetizers are sure to make an impression at any party.

**Ingredients**

- Cherry Tomatoes
- Horseradish
- Mayonnaise
- Fresh Herbs (your preference)

**Method**

1. Core the cherry tomatoes and scoop out centers. In a bowl, combine mayonnaise and horseradish to taste. Spoon mixture into tomatoes. Top with fresh herbs.

**Tomato Trivia**

*Combining tomatoes with fats (like mayonnaise, olive oil, or avocado) increases your absorption of the tomato's nutrients by 15%. Breastfeeding women should eat lots of tomato sauce to help their newborn get plenty of lycopene. The majority of the nutrients are housed in the tomato's skin so avoid peeling them.*

# 91. Salsa

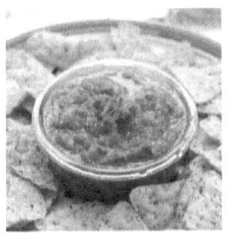

This isn't just any old salsa. Avocado and serrano chili provide unexpected and bold flavors.

**Ingredients**

- Tomatoes (diced)
- Corn Kernels
- Avocado (diced)
- Serrano Chili (minced)
- Cilantro (chopped)
- Salt to taste

**Method**

1. Combine all ingredients in a bowl. Mix well.

**Tomato Trivia**

*Coumaric acid and chlorogenic acid (found in tomatoes) protect your body from carcinogens (like pollution and smoke) so city dwellers and smokers alike should be eating tomatoes on the d daily. The vitamin A in tomatoes keeps your hair strong and glossy. It's also great for your teeth.*

# 92. Crunchy Tomatoes

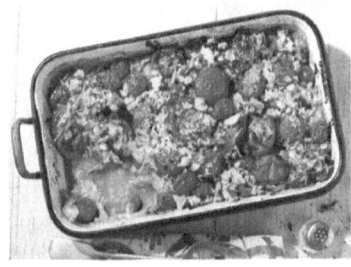

Replace your chips and popcorn with these delicious snacks.

**Ingredients**

- Tomatoes (sliced)
- Seasoned Breadcrumbs
- Olive Oil

**Method**

1. Arrange tomato slices in a pie dish. Pour in olive oil until partially submerged. Let soak 30 minutes. Turn slices over after 15 minutes. Remove from oil (save oil for salad dressing). Press one side of each slice into breadcrumbs.

**Tomato Trivia**

*Tomatoes that have green rings of unripe flesh around the stem are sweeter and more flavorful than the kind that are uniformly colored. Plum tomatoes are the most used for ketchups and sauces. Of the 7,500 species of tomato, only 13 of them are wild.*

### 93. Blue Cheese Tomato Salad

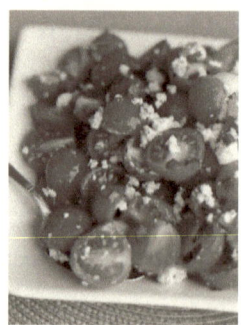

This salad is the perfect quick fix to any meal that's missing a side dish.

**Ingredients**

- Tomatoes (cut in wedges)
- Chives (chopped)
- Blue Cheese Dressing
- Pepper to taste

**Method**

1. Arrange tomato wedges on a platter. Drizzle blue cheese dressing over. Sprinkle chives and pepper on top.

**Tomato Trivia**

*To disprove the myth that tomatoes were poisonous, local New Jersey resident Robert Johnson ate an entire basket of them on the courthouse steps in 1820. After a childhood prank, Ronald Reagan didn't eat a single tomato for the next 70 years. Tomatoes are the key ingredient in 78% of America's most popular recipes.*

### 94. Chunky Tomato Basil Sauce

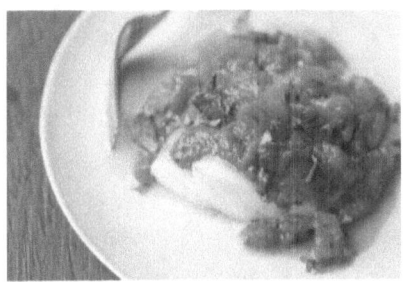

Use this sauce recipe to top pasta, fish, rice, polenta, or as a base for other sauces.

**Ingredients**

- 2 lbs. Cherry Tomatoes
- 7 cloves Garlic (sliced)
- 8 sprigs Basil
- 5 Tbsps. Olive Oil
- 1 Shallot (chopped)
- Salt & Pepper to taste

**Method**

1. Preheat oven to 350°F. Chop 1 lbs. tomatoes. Halve the other pound. Combine all ingredients in a large bowl with 4 tablespoons oil. Toss to coat. Line a baking sheet with 3 pieces of parchment paper. Spoon mixture on top of parchment. Fold paper over the mixture and crimp edges to seal. Bake 25-30 minutes (until saucy).

## Tomato Trivia

*The first recipe for spaghetti with tomato sauce dates back to 1790 by an Italian chef working in Russia. You can gauge nutrition value by color. The deeper the red, the more lycopene it contains. The smallest tomatoes are tomberries (less than 1" in diameter).*

### 95. Tomato Bread

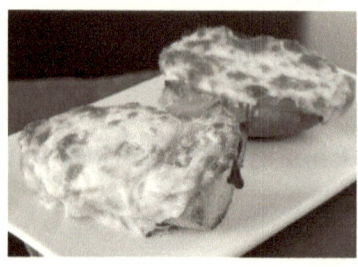

Say goodbye to plain old white bread and try out this rich, bold tomato bread with a touch of basil.

**Ingredients**

- 2 ½ cups Whole Grain Flour
- ¾ cup Warm Water
- 1 package Active Dry Yeast
- 3 Tbsps. Tomato Paste
- 2 Tbsps. Basil (dried)
- ¼ cup Parmesan Cheese (grated)
- 1 Tbsp. Sugar
- 1 Tbsp. Olive Oil
- 1 tsp Salt
- 1 tsp Crushed Red Pepper Flakes

**Method**

1. In a large bowl, dissolve yeast in warm water. Stir in basil, parmesan, sugar, salt, pepper flakes, tomato paste, oil, and 2 cups flour. Mix until combined. Add the rest of the flour 1 tablespoon at a time until a stiff dough is formed.

2. Knead on floured surface 3-5 minutes. Place in an oiled bowl. Cover with oiled plastic wrap. Let rise in a warm place until doubled in size. Punch dough down. Knead 1 minute. Shape into a loaf. Place on

greased baking sheet. Cover and let rise until doubled in size. Preheat oven to 375°F. Cut an X on the top of the loaf. Bake 40 minutes (or until golden).

**Tomato Trivia**

*While safe for humans, too many tomatoes can be toxic for dogs. They can be toxic to you as well, if eaten unripe (or if you eat the leaves and stems). But a puree of ripe tomatoes can help treat urinary tract infections.*

## 96. Tomato Cucumber Feta Salad

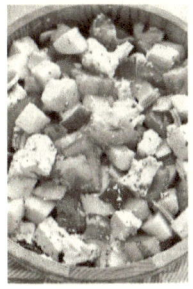

Add a refreshing and colorful side dish to your meal with this exquisitely simple salad.

**Ingredients**

- 2 lbs. Cucumber (chopped)
- 1 lbs. Tomatoes (chopped)
- 1 (7oz.) package Feta Cheese (crumbled)
- 1 bunch Scallions (chopped)
- 1 cup Olives (pitted, halved)
- ½ cup Fresh Mint (chopped)
- 6 Tbsps. Olive Oil
- ¼ cup Fresh Lemon Juice
- Salt & Pepper to taste

**Method**

1. Combine veggies and half of the feta in a large bowl. Mix in mint. In a small bowl, whisk together oil and lemon juice. Add salt and pepper. Pour dressing over salad. Toss to coat. Sprinkle remaining feta crumbles on top.

## Tomato Trivia

*The modern word for the fruit is almost identical in every language because they use a variation of the original Aztec "xitomatl." There are 4 species that stand out with the highest lycopene content: New Girl, Jet Star, Fantastic, and First Lady. There's no reason to spring for organic. Studies show that the species is more important than the method grown when it comes to nutrition.*

### 97. Tomato Matzo Balls

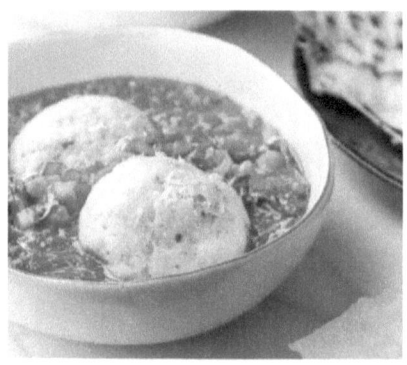

These rich matzo balls are perfect in a simple broth or covered in a creamy sauce.

## Ingredients

- 2 large Eggs
- 1 large Egg White
- 3 Tbsps. Tomato Paste
- ¾ cup Matzo Ball Mix
- 2 Tbsps. Olive Oil

## Method

1. Whisk together eggs and oil. Whisk in the tomato paste. Sprinkle in ½ cup matzo mix. Stir but mix as little as possible. Let chill in the fridge 20 minutes. Boil water.

2. Wet your hands in cold water. Scoop out a small ball (ping pong size) of the mixture with your hands. Disturb the mixture as little as possible. Gently form the lump into a ball. Reduce boiling water to a simmer. Drop balls into the simmering water. Simmer 20 minutes.

**Tomato Trivia**

*Tomatoes help prevent both constipation and diarrhea. Tomatoes contain phytonutrients that prevent blood clotting and lower bad cholesterol. New studies are showing that lycopene also prevents bone tissue from degrading.*

## 98. Tomato Marmalade

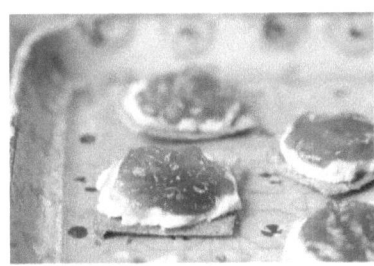

Spread this on toast, crackers, or pancakes for a sweet topping with a surprising note of tomato.

**Ingredients**

- 3 ½ lbs. Sweet Tomatoes
- 1 lbs. Lemons (seeded, sliced)
- 1 lbs. Oranges (seeded, sliced)
- 4 lbs. Sugar
- 4 oz. Fresh Lemon Juice
- 1 large pinch Saffron
- 1 Cinnamon Stick

**Method**

1. Place lemon and orange slices in a stainless-steel pot. Submerge in cold water. Place pot on high heat. Cover. Bring to a boil. Let boil 1 minute. Drain. Return slices to pot. Cover in 1" cold water. Bring to a boil over high heat. Reduce heat and simmer 35 minutes. Bring a pot of water to a boil. Drop the tomatoes in. Cook 1-2 minutes until skins loosen. Drain. Remove tomatoes skins. Use hands to tear tomatoes into chunks.

2. Place citrus and tomato in a glass or plastic container and refrigerate overnight. Pour mixture into a large preserving pan. Add cinnamon stick. Stir well. Bring to a boil over high heat. Cook 30 minutes or until it sets. Do not stir until it foams. Then, stir every few minutes. Marmalade is done when it looks glossy and contains tiny bubbles

throughout. Remove a small spoonful with a frozen spoon to check for a jelly consistency. Remove cinnamon stick. Pour marmalade into sterilized mason jars. Seal the jars.

**Tomato Trivia**

*Eat cooked tomatoes before bed. Lycopene improves sleep quality. Tomatoes are one of the few foods that can be used as both a fruit and a vegetable. In addition to versatility in the kitchen, tomatoes are also the base of many home remedies.*

## 99. Bacon Tomato Clams

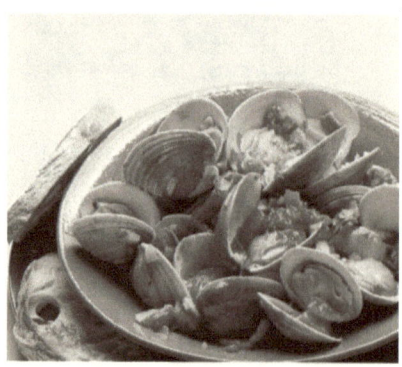

This unique dish creates a complex body of delicious flavors.

**Ingredients**

- 6 slices Bacon
- 1 (28oz.) can Diced Tomatoes
- 6 lbs. Clams
- ¼ cup Parsley
- 3 cloves Garlic
- 1 Onion (chopped)
- ½ cup Roasted Red Bell Peppers (from jar, drained)

**Method**

1. In a large pot on medium-high heat, add bacon and onions. Cook 8 minutes. Add garlic. Stir 1 minute. Add peppers and tomatoes with juice. Bring to a boil. Stir to combine. Add clams. Cover and boil 8-10 minutes, stirring occasionally. Stir in parsley. Serve.

**Tomato Trivia**

*A virgin Bloody Mary is an effective remedy for morning sickness. Gargling with tomato juice twice daily can treat mouth ulcers. Those with eczema or sun sensitivity should include tomato in every meal.*

## 100. Tomato Tarte Tatin

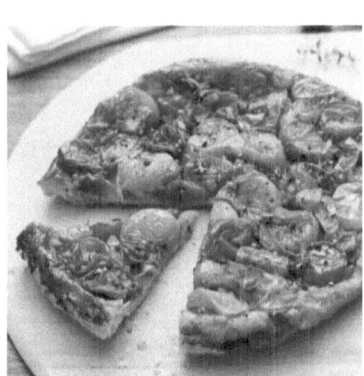

Finally treat tomato like the fruit it is with this exquisitely intriguing dessert.

**Ingredients**

- 1 ¾ lbs. Plum Tomatoes
- 1 sheet Puff Pastry
- ¾ cup Sugar
- 3 Tbsps. Butter (softened)
- 1 tsp Vanilla Extract
- Whipped Cream

**Method**

1. Preheat oven to 425°F. Boil water in a large pan. Drop in tomatoes. Cook 1 minute. Peel tomatoes. Core, halve, and remove seeds. Spread butter over bottom of large pan. Sprinkle in sugar.

2. Arrange tomatoes in single layer on top of butter. Place pan over medium heat. Cook 25 minutes, stirring occasionally. Remove from heat. Drizzle vanilla over tomatoes. Top with pastry rounds. Tuck in edges of pastry with knife. Cut 2-3 slits into each round. Bake until pastries are golden. Cook over medium heat for 10 minutes. Remove from pan onto platter.

## Tomato Trivia

*Place a slice of tomato on minor burns or wounds to soothe and heal them. 1-2 fresh tomatoes on an empty stomach can help reduce redness in the eyes. An ointment of tomato paste, lemon juice, and turmeric can be used as an effective treatment for dark circles.*

### 101. Polenta Gnocchi with Tomato Sauce

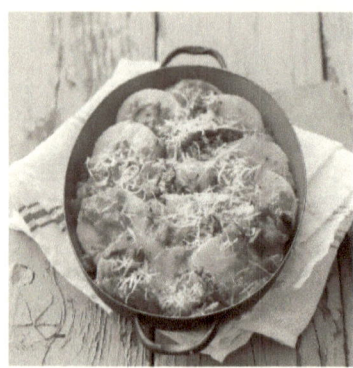

Polenta puts an interesting twist on this Gnocchi topped with a variation on the chunky sauce described earlier in this book.

### Ingredients

- Prepared Polenta
- Chunky Tomato Basil Sauce (see above)
- ½ cup Mushrooms (sliced)
- ¼ cup Parmesan (grated)
- Pepper to taste

### Method

1. Prepare chunky tomato basil sauce according to recipe. Line a baking sheet with aluminum foil. Grease with olive oil. Spread prepared polenta across in a smooth layer. Refrigerate 2-4 hours. Stamp out small polenta rounds.

2. Preheat oven to 400°F. Roll polenta into gnocchi shape. Grease a baking dish with olive oil. Arrange polenta rounds in dish so that they are slightly overlapping. Spoon in sauce generously. Bake 30 minutes. Remove from oven. Sprinkle with parmesan, parsley, and pepper.

**Tomato Trivia**

*Eat a blend of 6 oz. tomato paste with 3 cloves minced garlic as a remedy for diarrhea or infections (viral or bacterial). Drink tomato juice regularly if you're anemic. A facial mask made of tomato paste done weekly will minimize acne scars and reduce the number of breakouts.*

## 102. Tomato Watermelon Soup

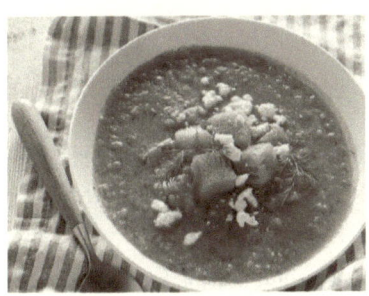

Tomato and watermelon combine to create a bold yet refreshing flavor in this soup.

### Ingredients

- 2 cups Watermelon (seeded, cubed)
- ½ lbs. Tomatoes (quartered)
- 2 Tbsps. Unsalted Almonds (ground)
- 1 Tbsp. Black Olives (pitted, chopped)
- 2 Tbsps. Feta (crumbled)
- 1 Tbsp. Fresh Lemon Juice
- 1 Tbsp. Red Wine Vinegar
- ½ Shallot (quartered)
- 2 tsp Fresh Mint
- 1 tsp Olive Oil

### Method

1. Pulse together all the ingredients (except feta, olives, and mint) in a food processor until smooth. Top with crumbled feta, olives, and mint.

**Tomato Trivia**

*Planting basil next to your tomatoes will increase your tomato yield by about 20%. Planting onions or garlic near your tomatoes will help ward off pests.*

*Tomatoes and Carrots are the best pals in the garden. They each strengthen the other.*

### 103. Tomato Terrine

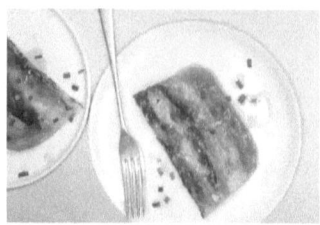

This summery dish is a perfect starter or light lunch on a hot afternoon.

**Ingredients**

- 6 lbs. Tomatoes (varying colors, peeled, quartered)
- 2 Carrots (chopped)
- 1 leek (sliced)
- 1 stalk Celery (chopped)
- 1 Shallot (halved)
- 1 clove Garlic
- 10 sprigs Parsley
- 10 Peppercorns
- 1 ½ Tbsps. Plain Gelatin
- ¼ cup Chives (sliced)
- 2 tsp Red Wine Vinegar
- 1 tsp Salt
- Olive Oil

**Method**

1. In a large pan, boil 3 cups of water with carrots, leeks, celery, shallots, garlic, parsley, peppercorns, and oil. Reduce heat to medium. Simmer 15 minutes. Strain through a fine sieve. Preserve liquid. Discard solids. Fillet the tomato wedges. Reserve the seeds and juice.

2. Press seeds and juice through fine sieve to collect ½ cup juice. Sprinkle the gelatin into the juice. Let stand 10 minutes. Add stock liquid from earlier. Whisk vigorously until gelatin dissolves. Stir in vinegar, salt, and chives. Pour into a greased baking dish that's lined with plastic wrap. Pour ½ cup liquid into pan. Chill 40 minutes.

3. Arrange 1-layer filleted tomato wedges on top of chilled liquid. Drizzle 2 tablespoons of liquid over them. Repeat these layers until ingredients are used up. Cover with plastic wrap. Weigh down the top with another pan with 2-3 heavy cans on top. Chill 6 hours.

**Tomato Trivia**

*The scientific name (solanum lycopersicum) meaning "wolf peach" comes from old werewolf myths in which this family of plants was used to transform into a werewolf. Throwing rotten tomatoes was a popular alternative to booing a bad performance in the 19$^{th}$ century. Indigo Rose, Sun Black and other purple or black tomatoes contain anthocyanin which is a powerful antioxidant.*

## BONUS: 27 SURPRISE RECIPES FOR SOMETHING DIFFERENT!

Making a tasty taco is not difficult. It is a quick and easy meal, however, sometimes it could be quite difficult to make it healthy. This BONUS section contains 27 awesome recipes for you to make light, but loaded (with flavor) tacos! It all depends on the ingredients that you are going to use and the way you are aiming to use these ingredients. For the light tacos, you should always prefer to choose the ingredients with low fats and low calories. For example, you can use white meat instead of beef or can use a vegetable sauce instead of cheese and cream.

Other than this, only choosing low fat and low-calorie ingredients is not enough. You should keep in view that how are you going to use them. For example, tortillas are one of the basic ingredients of tacos; so instead of flour or fried shells you should use the non-fried and steamed corn shells. If you need crispy shells, you can steam the tortillas to make them soft and then fold the shells. Finally, bake them for a few minutes at a high temperature in an oven. This is how you can cut out unnecessary fats and calories from your tacos. In short, keep in mind the impact of each ingredient of the finished meal. Check out these 27 recipes that focus on low calorie, low fat and high protein ingredients!

### 104. Taco Shells

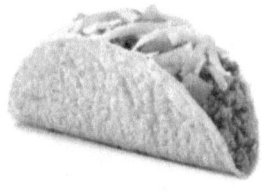

Taco shells are the basic ingredient of any taco recipe. It would be nice if you prepare the corn tortillas at home according to your own preference.

**Ingredients**

- Flour 2 cups
- Corn meal 1 cup
- Egg 2
- Water 3 cups
- Salt ½ tsp.

**Method**

1. Place flour in a shallow bowl. Beat eggs in another bowl. Add corn meal in flour and mix well. Make a well in the center of flour mixture. Fold in the eggs, water and salt and beat until you get smooth batter.

2. Heat up a griddle. (don't grease the griddle). Spoon 34 tbsp. of batter on hot griddle and spread it like a thinly pancake. When edges look dry then turn it over. (Don't let it brown). Let it dry on both side then shift them to cooling rack.

**Tips**

*The griddle should be ungreased. The batter should be smooth and lumps free. You can add the cumin seeds into the batter also. For low fats and diet tacos, don't fry taco shells. You should steam and bake the corn tortillas (taco shells).*

## 105. Taco with Wild Rice Filling

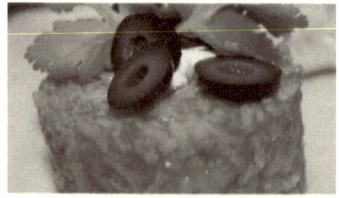

These tacos will be filled with organic grains; therefore, these tacos will be best for the person who prefers to eat a low sodium diet.

**Ingredients**

- Corn Taco Shells 5 shells
- Black beans ½ cup

- Organic Wild rice 1 cup
- Organic wild black barley ½ cup
- Brown Rice ½ cup
- Salt (optional) ¼ tsp.
- Chives 2 tbsp.
- Chili powder 1 tsp.
- Jalapeno (chopped) 3 medium size
- Salsa 2 tbsp.

**Method**

1. Steam tortilla shells (wrap them in the damp paper towel) in the preheated oven at 375 degrees Fahrenheit for 15 minutes. Then shift these tortillas to the oven rack and bake them for 10 minutes.

2. Take all other ingredients accept salsa and cook in ½ cup of water or until tender enough. Let the mixture cool (not much hot). Now take out corn tortillas from oven and fill with the Rice mixture. Top with salsa and serve. 2 servings can be made with it.

**Tips**

*I have listed salt as an optional ingredient because it tastes good with salt but you can skip it if you are using salsa. It is filled with the organic ingredients that are fiber rich and more notorious.*

### 106. Shrimp Taco

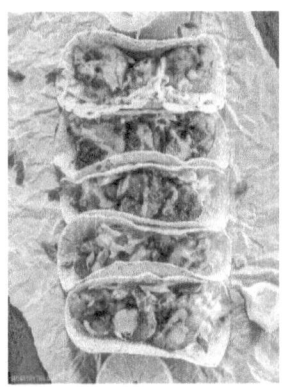

Shrimp is one of the most popular sea foods, and it's also quite healthy. Here's a great taco for all you seafood lovers.

## Ingredients

- Onion (diced) 1 small size
- Vegetable oil ½ cup
- Shrimps (cooked & chopped) 2 cups (1 pound)
- Taco shells 5 (medium size)
- Coriander leaves (diced ½ cup)
- Lime 1 small size
- Cabbage (diced) 1 cup
- Salt to taste

## Method

1. Steam and bake tortillas in oven. Now heat up oil in skillet and fry cabbage for 4 minutes. Add onions and cook for 3 minutes or until translucent. Add in shrimps and cook for 34 minutes. Now take out the tortillas and fill them with shrimp mixture. Sprinkle salt and lime juice. Sprinkle Coriander leaves and serve. 2 servings can be made.

## Tips

*Shrimps are one of the best sea food items. Anyone who is aimed at to take low calories diet, the Shrimp tacos are best for him. It is full of the nutrients but light, tasty and easy and quick to prepare.*

### 107. Chicken Tacos

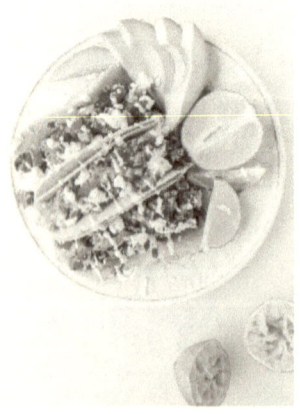

It is light, tasty and an easy recipe that anyone can enjoy it. It is full of flavor and nutrients.

## Ingredients

- Chicken Breast (boneless) 2 medium size
- Tomato paste ½ cup
- Lime juice 2 tbsp.
- Onion (diced ½ cup)
- Jalapeno (chopped) 1/4 cup
- Salt ¼ tsp.
- Roasted Red pepper (powder) ½ tsp.
- Vegetable oil ½ cup
- Corn tortilla shells (steamed and baked) 5 shells
- Water for cooking process

## Method

1. Cut the chicken breast into slices. Heat up oil in a deep skillet and add chicken slices to fry for 5 minutes. Stir in the tomato paste, salt, opinions and red chili powder and cook for other five minutes on medium heat. (Add 2 tbsp. water also). At last add jalapeno and a small amount of water. Keep it on low heat for 45 minutes. Sprinkle lemon juice. Now take steamed and baked tortilla shells and fill in with the chicken mixture. Now these are ready to serve. 2-3 servings can be made.

## Tips

*You can add other vegetables also. The chicken is one of the most popular white meat items. It is a low fat and heart friendly ingredient. If you use organic chicken (fed on natural food) it would be hundred times better than that of artificial food fed chicken.*

### 108. Bacon Tacos

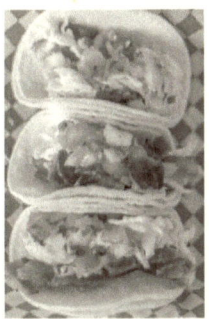

In bacon tacos, the Canadian bacon is used because it has fewer calories and fats, that's why, it will satisfy the hunger and will be nutritious also.

## Ingredients

- Canadian bacon 3 slices (medium size and thin)
- Chopped onions 1 cup
- Tomato paste 1 cup
- Broccoli (chopped) 1 cup
- Coriander leaves few leaves
- Red chili powder 1 tsp.
- Cumin ½ tsp.
- Vegetable oil 2 tbsp.
- Lime juice 2 tsp.
- Corn tortillas (steamed and baked) 3 shells

## Method

1. Boil and drain all vegetables. Now heat up oil in a pan and add cumin seeds in it. Now add all boiled veggies and chili powder and cook for 5 minutes. Take tortilla shells and place bacon slices in the shells. Then fill the shells with cooked vegetables. Sprinkle coriander leaves and lime juice and serve. 2-3 servings can be made.

## Tips

*You can also use American style bacon. You can use cabbage and carrot instead of broccoli but there is an amazing fact about broccoli that it supports the production of a particular enzyme that is helpful in protecting blood vessels.*

## 109. Spicy Ground Turkey Taco

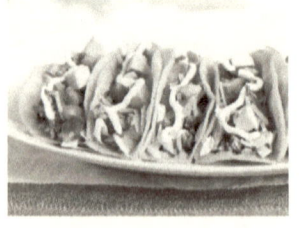

It is a delicious recipe with an amazing combination of meat and vegetables. It is a spicy recipe, so if you are making for kids then you can reduce the amount of spices.

**Ingredients**

- Lean ground turkey (extra lean) 1 cup
- Oregano 1 tsp.
- Chili powder 1 tsp.
- Roasted cumin ½ tsp.
- Coriander leaves (diced) 1 tsp.
- Lettuce (shredded) 1 and ½ cup
- Onion (chopped) ½ cup
- Tomato (diced) 2 medium size
- Jalapeno 2 (diced)
- Salsa 2 tbsp.
- Lime juice 2 tbsp.
- Corn tortillas (steamed and baked) 3 shells.

**Method**

1. In a nonstick frying pan cook the turkey and onions on medium heat. Add oregano, chili powder, cumin and 2 tbsp. water and mix well. Add tomatoes, lettuce and jalapeno and cook for 23 minutes. Fill the taco shells with turkey mixture and top with salsa and coriander leaves. Sprinkle lime juice and serve.

**Tips**

*Ground turkey is also rich in fats and calories, therefore while purchasing turkey for tacos, your choice should be turkey breast because it has lower fats and calories than dark meat. You should use extra lean turkey to control calories in your tacos.*

## 110. Tacos with Black Beans

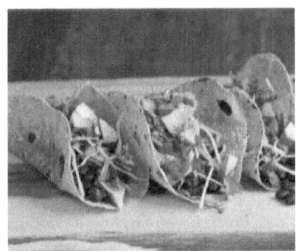

Black beans are one of the popular non-starchy vegetables. This recipe contains an amazing combination of vegetables.

**Ingredients**

- Black beans 1 cup
- Cabbage (shredded) ½ cup
- Onion (sliced) ½ cup
- Cheddar cheese (shredded) ¼ cup
- Avocado (peeled and sliced) ½ cup
- Chili powder ½ tsp.
- Green chilies (chopped) ¼ cup
- Salsa ½ cup
- Canola oil 2 tbsp.
- Taco shells (steamed and baked) 4 shells

**Method**

1. In a deep skillet sauté onions and cabbage in oil for few minutes. Add beans, chilies and salsa then bring to boil. Simmer for 5 minutes on low heat. Fill in taco shells with the mixture. Top with cheese and avocado and serve. 2 servings can be made.

**Tips**

*Soak the beans for 2 or 3 hours and then drain them before boiling. You can add salt to enhance the taste.*

### 111. Pinto Beans Taco

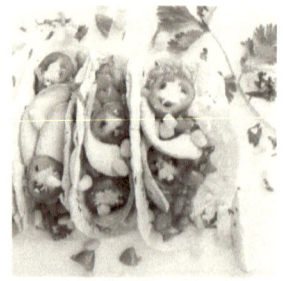

Pinto beans are full of fibers that are helpful for controlling the cholesterol level in your body. It is one of the most popular beans in the USA.

**Ingredients**

- Pinto beans (rinsed and drained) 1cup
- Vegetable oil 1 tbsp.

- Coriander (chopped) ½ cup
- Green chili (thin slices) ½ cup
- Tomato paste ½ cup
- Salt ¼ tsp.
- Tortilla shells (steamed and baked) 4 shells

**Method**

1. Heat up oil in a nonstick pan and add tomato paste in it. Then add salt and 1 tsp. coriander and cook for 1 minute. Fold in beans and cook for 58 minutes. Add 1 tbsp. lime juice and cook for two minutes. Fill the tortilla shells with beans mixture. Sprinkle green chili slices and coriander and serve. 2-3 servings can be made.

**Tips**

*Pinto beans are one of the heart friendly ingredients because these beans contain nutrients that are helpful for controlling cholesterol in human body. You can add other kinds of beans to enhance the flavor.*

## 112. Taco with Potato

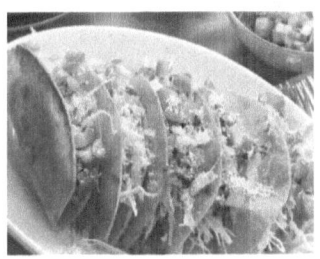

Potatoes are liked by everyone. From kids to old persons, there is great fan group for the potatoes in each age group. Taco with potatoes is a delicious recipe and anyone can enjoy it.

**Ingredients**

- Potatoes (boiled and mashed) 1 cup
- Cucumber (diced) 1 cup
- Salt 1 tsp.
- Green chili (chopped) ½ cup
- Tomatoes (chopped) ½ cup
- Corn tortillas (steamed and baked) 3 shells

**Method**

1. Place mashed potatoes in a bowl. Add salt and mix well. Now add half amount of chopped chilies and tomato and mix gently. Mix up cucumbers, remaining tomatoes and chilies in another bowl. Fill the taco shells with potato mixture. Then add the layer of cucumber mixture at the top and serve. 2-3 servings can be made.

**Tips**

*If you want to make these tacos lighter then reduce the amount of potatoes and add more vegetables like cabbage. Potatoes are helpful in lowering blood pressure because a potato contains a large amount of potassium that is a mineral which is helpful in lowering blood pressure and cholesterol in human body.*

### 113. Steamed Chicken Tacos

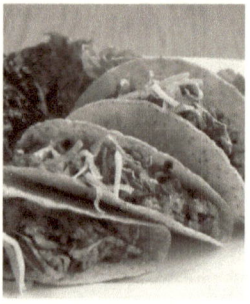

For steamed chicken tacos, you have to steam the chicken before proceeding to tacos. For this purpose, take a large amount of water in a large and deep pan. Add salt, garlic and ginger in water and bring to boil. Take 3 tbsp. lemon juice, add ½ tsp. salt and 2 tbsp. garlic paste and mix well. Grease the chicken with lemon mixture.

Now place the chicken on a small wire stand (that can be placed in the pot of water) and place in the boiling water. Cover the pot for 1 hour. Now remove the cover and check if the chicken is translucent then take it out, if not, then keep in for more time.

**Ingredients**

- Boneless steamed chicken (small cubes) 1 and ½ cup
- Jalapeno (chopped) 4 medium size
- Roasted cumin 2 tsp.

- Black pepper powder ¼ tsp.
- Boiled black beans 2 tbsp.
- Tomato paste 1 cup
- tomatoes (chopped) ½ cup
- Canola oil 2 tbsp.
- Taco shells (steamed and baked) 2 shells.

**Method**

1. Heat up oil in a nonstick frying pan. Add tomato paste, cumin and black pepper powder and cook for few minutes. Add black beans and jalapeno and cook for few minutes. Spoon tomato mixture in the taco shells then fill with chicken. Spoon another layer of tomato mixture. Top with chopped tomatoes and serve.

**Tips**

*You can use steamer for steaming chicken. Chicken is a low calories and low fats ingredient; especially chicken breast. Therefore, try to use boneless chicken breast pieces.*

### 114. Tofu Tacos

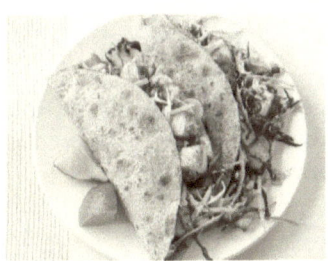

It is a unique and amazing taco recipe that requires baked tofu for filling. It is an easy and quick recipe.

**Ingredients**

- Firm Tofu (cubes) 1 cup
- Egg (beaten) 1 large size
- All-purpose flour 1 cup
- Bread crumbs ½ cup
- Cabbage (shredded) ½ cup
- Taco shells (steamed and baked) 4 shells

**Method**

1. Prepare a baking sheet and preheat the oven at 375 degrees. Place flour in a bowl and beaten egg in another bowl. Drain the tofu cubes with paper towel to make them dry.

2. Now dip tofu cubes in all-purpose flour and then in eggs. Then roll these cubes in bread crumbs and place on prepared baking sheet. Bake the tofu cubes for 810 minutes in preheated oven. Then take out and turn over all cubes then bake again for 810 minutes. Now fill the taco shells with tofu cubes and cabbage. Now it is ready to serve.

**Tips**

*Tofu is made by soybean curd. It is a gluten free ingredient and rich in iron, calcium and dietary protein.*

### 115. Taco with Roasted Vegetables

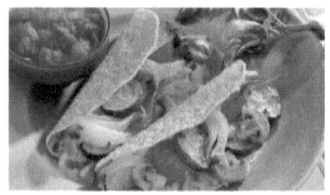

This recipe calls for vegetables that should be roasted. You can use your desirable vegetables for your tacos. Here we are enlisting the light tacos so be careful about the choice of vegetables.

**Ingredients**

- Onion (chopped) 1 cup
- Red bell pepper (seedless) 1 cup
- Zucchini (chopped) ½ cup
- Garlic powder ½ tsp.
- Carrots (diced) ½ cup
- Black pepper powder ¼ tsp.
- Sea salt ¼ tsp.
- Cumin ½ tsp.
- Vegetable oil ¼ cup
- Lime juice 2 tbsp.
- Corn tortillas (steamed and baked) 5 shells

**Method**

1. Prepare a baking sheet and preheat the oven at 400 degrees. Toss all vegetables in oil. Then place all vegetable on baking sheet and sprinkle cumin salt and pepper on them. Roast the vegetables for 1015 minutes. Then take out the vegetable, rearrange the vegetables and roast again for 10 minutes. Fill the taco shells with roasted vegetables and sprinkle lime juice. Now the tacos are ready to shells. 2-3 servings can be made.

**Tips**

*You can use vegetable sauce for it. Tomato or chili sauce will be a good addition for this recipe. You should try to use non-starchy vegetables for this recipe but can add small amount of your favorite starchy vegetable.*

### 116. Meat Ball Taco

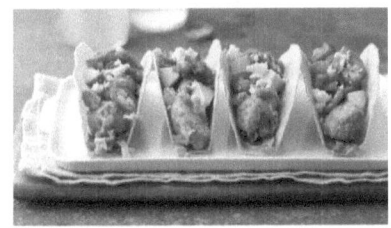

Meat balls can be cooked by using any meat but I have used turkey meat for low calories.

**Ingredients**

- Ground turkey 1 pound
- Egg 1 large size
- Evaporated milk 1 cup
- Vegetable soup (condensed) 1 cup
- Bread crumbs ½ cup
- Cucumber (chopped) ½ cup
- Tomatoes (chopped) ½ cup
- Green chili (chopped) ¼ cup
- Corn tortillas (steamed and baked) 5 shells

**Method**

1. In a shallow bowl place meat, beaten egg and breadcrumbs and mix well. Make small balls of 1 inch. Heat up skillet on medium heat. Cook

the meat ball until all sides are brown. Add milk and vegetable soup and cook for 12-15 minutes. Fill the taco shell with meat ball mixture. Mix up tomatoes, cucumber and cucumbers in a bowl. Add a layer of vegetable mixture on meatball filling. Serve hot. 4 servings can be made.

**Tips**

*For making you tacos lighter you can reduce the amount of meat balls and can add more vegetables for filling.*

### 117. Egg Taco

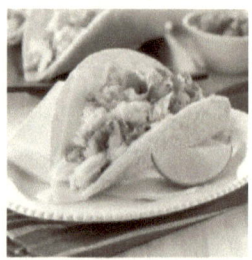

This recipe calls for hard boiled eggs with vegetable sauces. It is quick, easy and delicious recipe. Anyone can prepare it at home.

**Ingredients**

- Hard boiled eggs 4 eggs
- Boiled carrots (chopped) 2 cups
- Green beans (boiled) 1 cup
- Green chili (diced) ¼ cups
- Salt to taste
- Lettuce 3 leaves
- Vegetable sauce ½ cup
- Tortillas (steamed and baked) 3 shells

**Method**

1. Cut the boiled eggs in round shape (like cookies). In a bowl mix up gently eggs slices, boiled carrots, beans and green chili. Sprinkle a small amount of salt and mix carefully. Spoon the egg mixture on lettuce leaves and wrap it. Put each filled lettuce leaves in taco shells for filling.

## Tips

*Eggs are rich in Vitamin A. Therefore, the use eggs save a person from blindness. The green beans are rich in Vitamin B1 and useful minerals like phosphorus, calcium etc.*

## 118. Baked Cauliflower Tacos

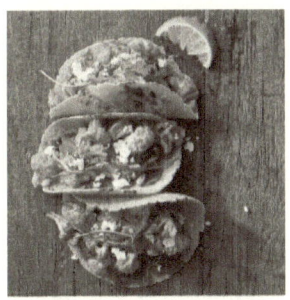

This is an amazing recipe that is not only tasty but is also low in calories. You will not feel bloated after eating these tacos.

**Ingredients**

- Cauliflower 2 cups
- Bread crumbs 1 cup
- Mustered 1 tbsp.
- Marinara sauce ¼ cup
- Egg 1 egg
- Taco mix ½ tbsp.
- Sea salt to taste
- Black pepper to taste
- Corn tortilla (steamed and baked) 2 shells

**Method**

1. Beat the egg in shallow bowl. Add mustered powder and beat again to mix well. In another bowl mix up breadcrumbs and taco mix. Prepare a baking sheet and preheat the oven at 375 degrees.

2. Now dip each cauliflower floret in the egg mixture then coat with breadcrumbs mixture. Spread all florets on prepared baking sheet and bake for 15 18 minutes or until golden brown. Fill the taco shells with cauliflower florets and then spread hot marinara sauce on it.

**Tips**

*You can use your desirable sauce for seasoning and can add other vegetables like tomatoes, chili, cabbage etc.*

## 119. Roasted Mushrooms Tacos

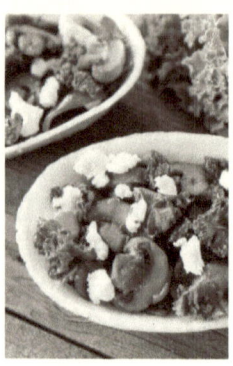

It is not only a mouthwatering recipe but nutritious and healthy also.

**Ingredients**

- Mushrooms 10 pieces
- Minced garlic 1 tbsp.
- Parmesan cheese (grated) 1/2 cup
- Black pepper (grated) ¼ tsp.
- Onion powder 1 tbsp.
- Vegetable oil 2 tbsp.
- Tomato (chopped) ½ cup
- Lime juice 1 tbsp.
- Tortillas (steamed and baked) 4 shells

**Method**

1. Preheat the oven at 375 degrees and prepare a baking sheet. Heat up oil in a nonstick skillet and add mushrooms and garlic. Cook until no runny juice left. Let it cool. Meanwhile mix up cheese, black pepper and add it to the mushrooms and mix gently.

2. Spread mushrooms on baking sheet and bake for 20 minutes. Fill each shell with baked mushrooms and spread chopped tomatoes at mushrooms and serve.

**Tips**

*Mushrooms are low calories ingredient that are likes in all part s of world. A mushroom contains iron and vitamin D that are most important for strong bones.*

## 120. Taco with Stir Fry Vegetables

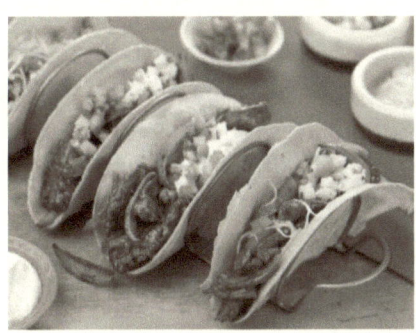

This taco recipe is really awesome. It contains a great combination of vegetables that is not only eye catching, but rich in taste and nutrition also.

**Ingredients**

- Broccoli florets 1 cup
- Cauliflower florets ½ cup
- Carrots (small finger slices) ½ cup
- Mushrooms (sliced) ½ cup
- Baby corns (cut in 4 pieces)
- Green and red chili (chopped) ½ cup
- Water ¼ cup
- Salt to taste
- Olive oil 2 tbsp.
- Desirable vegetable sauce 1 cup
- Corn tortillas (steamed and baked) 4 shells

**Method**

1. Heat up oil (until smoke) in a large frying pan. Add all vegetables and stir and cook for few minutes. Add water and salt and cook until all vegetables are tender and crispy and water free. Fill taco shells and sprinkle pepper and lime juice for seasoning. Top with desirable vegetable sauce and serve.

## Tips

*Broccoli and cauliflower help to reduce cholesterol therefore it is best for people who are suffering from high cholesterol. These vegetables are heart friendly because the high cholesterol is one of the basic reasons of heart diseases.*

### 121. Taco with Mexican Salsa

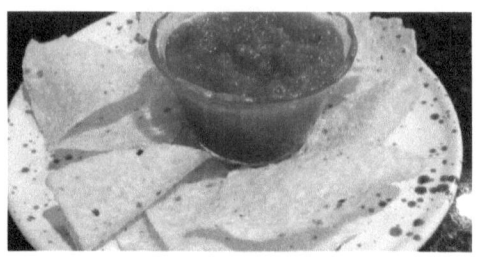

In this recipe, you get a great combination of boiled chicken and salsa. It is best for spring lunches.

### Ingredients

- Boiled chicken (boneless cubes) 1 ½ cup
- Tomatoes (chopped) 1 cup
- Onion (chopped) ½ cup
- Jalapeno ¼ cup
- Cilantro ½ cup
- Lime Juice ¼ cup
- Black pepper (grinded) 1 tsp.
- Salt to taste
- Garlic cloves (minced) ¼ tsp.
- Dill (fresh) 1 tbsp.
- Red wine vinegar 1 tbsp.
- Plain yogurt 1 cup
- Corn tortilla shells (steamed and baked) 4 shells

### Method

1. Place yogurt in a bowl and add garlic, dill, red wine vinegar and black pepper and mix well. In another bowl place all remaining vegetables and mix gently. Sprinkle salt and lime juice and mix gently until all vegetables get coated with lime juice.

2. Take taco shells and place a layer of boiled chicken in each shell for filling. Then add a layer of yogurt mixture and then a layer of vegetable mixture in each taco shells. Now the tacos are ready to serve.

**Tips**

*You can replace yogurt sauce with tomato sauce or any other desirable sauce.*

### 122. Minced Chicken Tacos

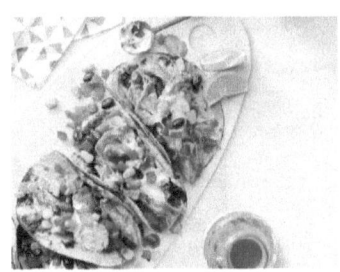

The minced chicken is used in this recipe. The minced chicken is easy to cook and easy to digest. You should use the chicken breast because this part of chicken contains least amount of fats.

**Ingredients**

- Minced chicken 2 cups
- Onion (diced) ½ cup
- Tomato paste 1 cup
- Green chili (diced) ¼ cup
- Salt to taste
- Vegetable sauce 1 cup
- Coriander leaves (diced) ¼ cup
- Vegetable oil 3 tbsp.
- Corn taco shells 3 shells

**Method**

1. Heat up oil in a nonstick frying pan. Add chicken and cook for 3 minutes. Add onion and cook for 5 minutes. Add tomato paste and cook for 5 minutes on low heat. Add chili and cover the pan and reduce the heat. Let it cook for 8-10 minutes. Fill the taco shells with chicken mixture and desirable vegetable sauce. Sprinkle coriander leaves and serve.

**Tips**

*You can use small chicken cubes to replace the minced chicken. The cabbage and cucumber can be a good addition to the recipe. Cucumber helps the digestion process.*

### 123. Stir Fry Shrimp Taco

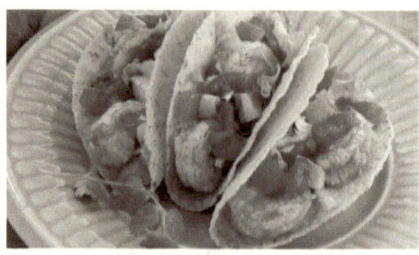

Shrimps are one of the most popular ingredients of sea food. The combination of shrimp and chicken broth tastes excellent.

**Ingredients**

- Shrimps (peeled and deveined) 1 pound
- Chicken broth (reduced sodium) 1 cup
- Rice vinegar 1 tbsp.
- Red pepper powder 1 tsp.
- Carrots (thinly sliced) ½ cup
- Cabbage (chopped) 2 cups
- Green onion (thinly sliced) ¼ cup
- Canola oil 2 tbsp.
- Sesame oil 2 tsp.
- Soy sauce (reduced sodium) 2 tbsp.
- Corn starch 1 tbsp.
- Corn tortillas (steamed and baked) 5 shells

**Method**

1. Mix up corn starch and broth in a bowl. Add soy sauce, vinegar and sesame oil and mix well. Heat up canola oil in a nonstick pan. Stir fry the shrimps for a minute. Add chili powder and fry until shrimps are pink. Take out shrimps and now fry carrots in it for few minutes.

2. Stir in corn starch and broth mixture and bring to boil (cook until thickened). Add onion, peas and cabbage and cook for 2 minutes. Add

shrimp mixture and cook for few seconds. Fill taco shells with the stir fry shrimp mixture and serve.

**Tips**

*Shrimps are considered one of the world's healthiest foods. The shrimp are good for brain health and bones. They support red blood cells that provide oxygen to the body.*

### 124. Stir Fry Chicken Taco

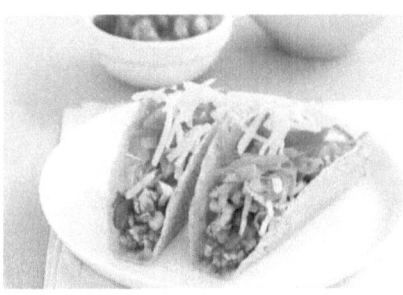

This recipe calls for mushrooms and vegetable with chicken. Therefore, it contains a great combination of healthy ingredients.

**Ingredients**

- Bone less chicken breast (1/2-inch cubes) 2 cups
- Onion (thin wedges) ½ cup
- Green beans 1 cup
- Red bell pepper (sliced) ¼ cup
- Mushrooms (sliced) 1 cup
- Vegetable broth 1/4 cup
- Garlic (minced) ¼ tsp.
- Sesame oil 1 tbsp.
- Soy sauce 3 tbsp.
- Canola oil 3 tbsp.
- Corn tortillas (steamed and baked) 4 shells

**Method**

1. Heat up oil in a nonstick pan. Add chicken and cook for 45 minutes. Add onion and fry for 2 minutes. Add mushrooms and red bell pepper and cook for few minutes. In a bowl mix up and blend the sauce ingredients and add in to chicken mixture and cook for few minutes.

Add green beans and broth and bring to boil. Cook until thickened. Fill taco shells with the mixture and serve hot.

## Tips

*It would be great to use the rich mineral vegetable broth, because it is cost effective and health friendly ingredient. You can use different types of mushrooms like button mushrooms, wild mushrooms etc.*

### 125. Roasted Chicken Tacos

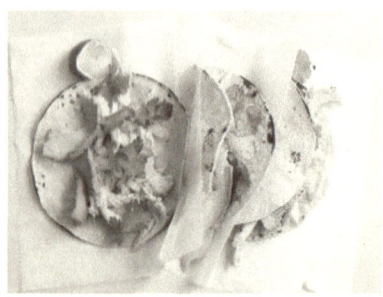

This recipe calls for chicken with garlic. Garlic is one the most popular ingredients of Asian recipes.

## Ingredients

- Chicken breast (boneless, cut in halves) 4 pieces
- Butter 3 tbsp.
- Garlic powder 2 tsp.
- Onion powder 2 tbsp.
- Salt ½ tsp.
- Tomato (diced) ½ cup
- Coriander - few leaves
- Green chili (diced) ¼ tsp.
- Tortillas (steamed and baked) 4 shells

## Method

1. Heat up butter in a skillet and bring to melt. Coat chicken pieces with salt, garlic and onion powder. Add chicken in butter and sauté it for 10-18 minutes from all sides or until juice is run out.

2. Blend tomatoes, coriander leaves and green chili (with a splash of salt) in the blender until smooth. Cut the cooked chicken pieces into finger

shape slices. Fill the taco shells with chicken slices. Then add a layer of tomato sauce on them and serve.

## Tips

*You can use fish to replace the chicken or can use both together. It really tastes great with the combination of fish and chicken. But the amount of fish should be less than the amount of chicken. You can add lime juice to enhance the flavor.*

### 126. Wild Mushroom Taco

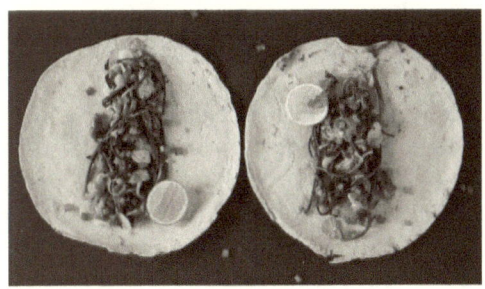

This is a light and tasty recipe that is also quick and easy to make.

## Ingredients

- Wild mushrooms (chopped) 1 ½ cup
- Button mushrooms (sliced) 1 cup
- Vegetable oil 1 tbsp.
- Soy butter 1 tbsp.
- Tomato paste 2 tbsp.
- Mustered powder ¼ tsp.
- Salt to taste
- Black and red pepper powder ½ tsp. each
- Onion (diced) ½ cups
- Taco shells (steamed and baked) 3 shells

## Method

1. Heat up oil and butter in a pan. Add onion and cook until light brown. Add garlic and cook for 2 minutes. Add mushrooms and tomato paste and sauté for few minutes. Add mustered powder and pepper powder and cook for few minutes. Fill taco shells and serve with desirable sauce.

## Tips

*You can add vegetables like cucumber, carrots and cabbage to the filling. You can add 1 tbsp. cream also.*

### 127. Minced Beef Tacos

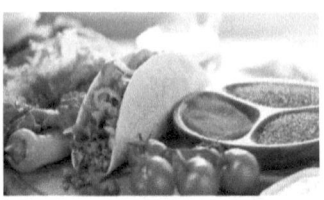

This recipe calls for minced beef that is rich in fats and cholesterol. That's why you should use small amount of beef and vegetables.

## Ingredients

- Minced beef (boiled) ½ cup
- Green beans (boiled) 1 cup
- Spinach (boiled and mashed) ½ cup
- Tomato paste 1 cups
- Vegetable oil 2 tbsp.
- Green chili (chopped) ½ cup
- Cabbage (chopped) 1 ½ cup
- Lime juice 2 tsp.
- Tortilla shells (steamed and baked) 4 shells

## Method

1. Heat up oil in a pan. Add tomato paste and cook for 3 minutes. Add salt and spinach and cook for few minutes. Add minced beef and cook for 5 minutes. Add green beans and chili. Cook for few minutes or until no runny liquid left. Fill taco shells with the beef mixture. Sprinkle lime juice then add a layer of cabbage and serve.

## Tips

*The beef contains large amount of fats and calories, so before using minced beef, it is better to boil the beef in large amount of water then drain it. In this way you will be able to reduce the fats and calories of beef. You can that water as broth for another recipe.*

## 128. Taco with Green Filling

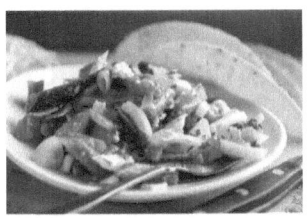

This recipe contains green ingredients like spinach, green beans, coriander, etc., for filling. It tastes great with lime juice and cauliflower.

**Ingredients**

- Spinach (boiled and mashed) 1 cup
- Green beans (boiled) 1 cup
- Oregano ¼ cup
- Coriander leaves (diced) ¼ cup
- Tomato paste ¼ cup
- Green chili (diced) ¼ cup
- Cauliflower florets ½ cup
- Broccoli florets 1 ½ cup
- Vegetable oil 3 tbsp.
- Salt to taste
- Black pepper powder ¼ tsp.
- Onion powder 1 tbsp.
- Water ½ cup.
- Cabbage (chopped) 1 cup
- Tomato (chopped) ½ cup
- Cucumber (sliced) ½ cup
- Tortillas (steamed and baked) 4 shells

**Method**

1. Combine spinach, coriander and oregano and blend them with tomato paste. Heat up 1 tbsp. oil in a pan then add spinach mixture, 2 tbsp. water and a splash of salt and cook on medium heat for 5 minutes. Take remaining water in another pan, add salt, black pepper powder and onion powder and place on medium. Bring the water to boil and add cauliflower and broccoli florets in it. Cook until florets are translucent.

2. Take the florets out and heat up remaining oil in a pan and fry the florets for few minutes. Fill the taco shells with fried florets and the spread a

layer of spinach sauce on it. Spread cucumber, tomato and cabbage at the top and serve.

**Tips**

*This recipe includes spinach that is full of Iron and is helpful for maintaining bowl movements. Other than this, the green ingredients are usually rich in vitamin C.*

### 129. Egg Potato Taco

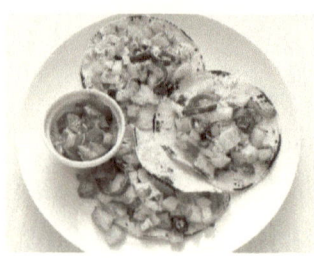

Eggs are full of Vitamin A. The deficiency of Vitamin A affects eye sight and causes blindness and it is a very common deficiency that is observed in the kids.

**Ingredients**

- Potato (boiled and peeled) ½ cup
- Egg (boiled and sliced) 1 cup
- Black pepper ¼ cups
- Cabbage (chopped) 1 cup
- Tomato sauce ½ cup
- Corn tortillas (steamed and baked) 3 shells

**Method**

1. Cut the boiled potatoes in small cubes. Add cabbage egg slices and mix gently. Add black pepper and mix gently. Fill taco shells with the mixture and spread tomato sauce on filling. Now it is ready to serve.

**Tips**

*You can add yams to replace potatoes and can use chili sauce also. If you want to make the potatoes crispy then coat them with butter and bake for few minutes, but for making them crispy don't cut them in cubes but in slices.*

## 130. Corn Chicken Tacos

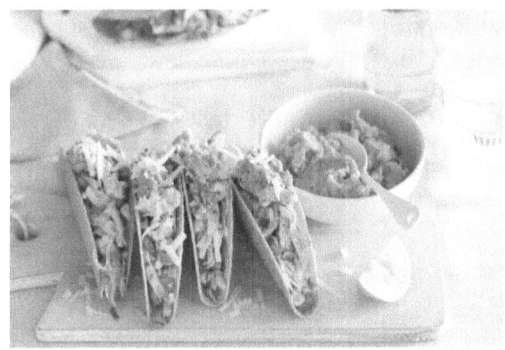

This is a spicy and mouthwatering recipe; especially for those who love to eat spicy food.

**Ingredients**

- Chicken (small boneless cubes) 1 cup
- Red bell pepper x2
- Green chili (diced) ¼ cup
- Vegetable oil 3 tbsp.
- Tomato paste 1 tbsp.
- Corn seeds (boiled) ½ cup
- Salt to taste
- Cucumber (diced) ½ cup
- Lime juice 2 tbsp.
- Tortillas (steamed and baked) 3 shells

**Method**

1. Heat up oil in a pan and add tomato paste, salt and red bell pepper. Cook for 3 minutes. Add chicken, corn seeds and lime juice. Cook for five minutes. Spread green chili and cover pan for few minutes. Reduce heat and cook for 34 minutes. Fill taco shells with chicken mixture and spread cucumber on filling and serve.

**Tips**

*Corn is helpful for controlling diabetes and heart diseases. In short, it is a heart friendly and health friendly ingredient that not only fuel the body but save it from heart diseases and diabetes.*

## Final Words

I would like to thank you for downloading my book and I hope I have been able to help you and educate you about something new.

**If you have enjoyed this book and would like to share your positive thoughts, could you please take 30 seconds of your time to go back and give me a review on my Amazon book page!**

**I greatly appreciate seeing these reviews because it helps me share my hard work!**

Again, thank you and I wish you all the best with your cooking journey!

# Last Chance to Get YOUR Bonus!

**FOR A LIMITED TIME ONLY** – Get Olivia's best-selling book *"The #1 Cookbook: Over 170+ of the Most Popular Recipes Across 7 Different Cuisines!"* absolutely FREE!

Readers have absolutely loved this book because of the wide variety of recipes. It is highly recommended you check these recipes out and see what you can add to your home menu!

Once again, as a big thank-you for downloading this book, I'd like to offer it to you *100% FREE for a LIMITED TIME ONLY!*

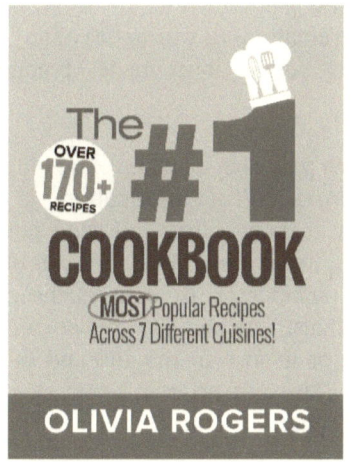

## Get your free copy at:

# TheMenuAtHome.com/Bonus

## Disclaimer

This book and related site provides recipe and food advice in an informative and educational manner only, with information that is general in nature and that is not specific to you, the reader. The contents of this book and related site are intended to assist you and other readers in your personal efforts. Consult your physician or nutritionist regarding the applicability of any information provided in our information to you.

Nothing in this book should be construed as personal advice or diagnosis, and must not be used in this manner. The information provided about conditions is general in nature. This information does not cover all possible uses, actions, precautions, side-effects, or interactions of medicines, or medical procedures. The information in this site should not be considered as complete and does not cover all diseases, ailments, physical conditions, or their treatment.

**No Warranties:** The authors and publishers don't guarantee or warrant the quality, accuracy, completeness, timeliness, appropriateness or suitability of the information in this book, or of any product or services referenced by this site.

The information in this site is provided on an "as is" basis and the authors and publishers make no representations or warranties of any kind with respect to this information. This site may contain inaccuracies, typographical errors, or other errors.

**Liability Disclaimer:** The publishers, authors, and other parties involved in the creation, production, provision of information, or delivery of this site specifically disclaim any responsibility, and shall not be held liable for any damages, claims, injuries, losses, liabilities, costs, or obligations including any direct, indirect, special, incidental, or consequences damages (collectively known as "Damages") whatsoever and howsoever caused, arising out of, or in connection with the use or misuse of the site and the information contained within it, whether such Damages arise in contract, tort, negligence, equity, statute law, or by way of other legal theory.

www.ingramcontent.com/pod-product-compliance
Lightning Source LLC
Chambersburg PA
CBHW031119080526
44587CB00011B/1037